A DOCTOR RETIRES—
IS THERE LIFE AFTER MEDICINE?

A DOCTOR RETIRES—
IS THERE LIFE AFTER MEDICINE?

Orel Friedman, M.D.

To order additional copies of this book, contact:
Xlibris Corporation
1-888-795-4274
www.Xlibris.com
Orders@Xlibris.com
26741

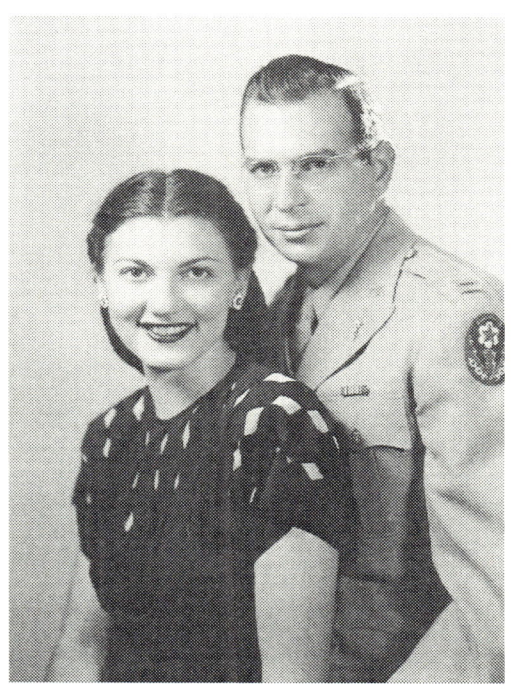

To my late wife, Blossom, a woman of valor

A woman of valor who can find?
For her price is far above rubies.
The heart of her husband doth safely trust in her,
And he hath no lack of gain.
She doeth him good and not evil
All the days of her life

Proverbs 31:10-12

PART I

Chapter 1

While driving my wife and friends to a dinner party, the car in front of me suddenly appeared like two identical cars, one above the other. As an experienced physician, I reflexly closed one eye to see if the double vision disappeared. It did and reappeared with both eyes open.

Concerned but knowing it would be safe to drive with one eye closed, nothing was said about the problem; and in a few minutes, our destination was reached. Although relieved for the moment, instinctively, I knew this meant trouble without realizing that soon my life as a medical practitioner would be ended forever.

There was no problem during the evening, but I asked my wife to drive us home where I described the double vision episode to her.

During the next few days, which were over a weekend, my professional activities were not affected, but occasionally, there was transitory double vision. This seemed to be increasing along with my concern and apprehension.

This led to an emergency appointment with my ophthalmologist. He confirmed that there was a definite eye-muscle imbalance leading to the double vision.

Since this condition was not transitory and most likely would get worse, I decided to immediately cancel all scheduled surgery. Hopefully, I could continue my otolaryngology (ear, nose, and throat) and allergy office practice while undergoing studies to try to determine the underlying cause of my visual problem.

The wisdom of this approach was never questioned since it was not my nature to consider performing surgery as an impaired physician. However, it was traumatic to cancel all my scheduled surgery and refer my patients to my colleagues.

Immediately, a search for an ear, nose, and throat specialist to come in and help continue my practice was begun. It was the month of April when no residents were finishing their training and becoming available. No one was found immediately or for the next month. My frustration mounted with the increasing difficulty trying to keep my office practice going since it included an active allergy practice with patients coming in regularly for injections.

Medically, I had a CAT scan and various consultations. The causal diagnosis was that the severe hyperthyroidism I had suffered the year before with extensive muscle atrophy led to a considerable aggravation of a lifelong minimal eye-muscle imbalance when the atrophied muscles healed. Consultations were held with two eye-muscle specialists at two medical schools. The first consultant recommended immediate corrective surgery.

The other advised a conservative approach during which eye strain was to be avoided. From my personal experience at this time, being conservative seemed reasonable because my vision was quite good in the morning. However, after several hours examining patients, the double vision would become persistent. Hopefully, my vision would stabilize with rest, and then corrective lenses would provide the solution. I decided against having surgery performed at the time.

An additional problem was with my employees. My nurse had left a couple of weeks before, and no one had been found to replace her. My full-time secretary, a single mother who needed to work, had been offered a very good position at our hospital. Under normal circumstances, she would have turned it down because of loyalty to me. The other offer had to be decided upon without delay. She had to make a quick decision, and realizing that the instability caused by my problem might soon leave her unemployed, she very regretfully and tearfully gave me two weeks' notice that she was leaving.

All these upsetting developments occurred in the two weeks since I first noted my double vision. The thought was overwhelming that in two more weeks, all the office assistance available would be a part-time secretary and my wife who filled in as a receptionist in emergencies. Also, because I was not performing surgery, I had more time to spend in my office and was seeing more patients than usual which was becoming stressful.

I pondered and agonized. What could I and should I do under the circumstances? My wife understood my dilemma and was very supportive. I respected her wisdom and judgment and sought her advice. We had a long, frank, and meaningful discussion about my ability to continue working with my disability. After all, I had a well-established, excellent reputation, and in no way did I want to endanger or spoil it.

The welfare of my patients was always foremost in my mind and practice. It was obvious that no competent physician in my field was available to help me. I was unable to operate and probably never would again. To try to find and train new office personnel in the next two weeks was beyond my staff's capacity and mine. My office would be in chaos without competent assistants. Trying to conduct an office practice was aggravating my double vision and daily becoming more stressful. Under these circumstances, my vision would not improve.

My future looked bleak and impossible. We agreed that I had no choice but to close my office and quit the practice of medicine.

This meant a precipitous drop in my income, and we discussed the present and future implications of this action. Fortunately, I had taken out disability insurance many years before. I asked my ophthalmologist if he would certify that I was disabled if I quit working. There was no question in his mind about my disability and agreed to do all the paperwork necessary to support my claim.

With the insurance problem settled, I told my wife and my office staff that I would wind down my practice and close my office in two weeks. It was a bittersweet decision. I was relieved that an impossible struggle would soon be over, but I was not prepared for retirement at age, sixty-six.

Chapter 2

At almost any other time, my wife, who was extremely capable, would have stepped in and done a full day's work in this crisis to help me out. However, she was the president of the Upstate Region of Hadassah, a very responsible and time-consuming position as a volunteer. Hadassah is a Jewish women's service organization.

Their annual regional conference was scheduled to be held in Utica, New York, the first week in May, which coincided with the week when my secretary would no longer be working in my office.

My wife was very busy writing speeches, making final arrangements, and preparing for the conference. Under no circumstances could or would I ask her to give up this crowning organizational moment of her life because I needed her help. She was encouraged to continue her own efforts, but at the same time, it represented another inescapable roadblock to my continuing.

My determination to close my office in two weeks was dictated by the realization that once my secretary left, it would be impossible to maintain the high standards I demanded of myself and my office staff. Over the years, I had observed people in all walks of life who had held on too long, not knowing when to quit, and the ruinous consequences of their actions. My long-established mind-set was to let go when the time came, and if I erred, it would be too early rather than too late. For me, the time had come, and no matter how excruciating, I was going to quit.

The two weeks were harrowing, and the time much too short, but everyone in the office worked very hard to make the transition as smooth as possible.

My colleagues in the same specialty, who already had cooperated in taking over my surgical patients, were immediately informed of my decision. All the other physicians were notified by a form letter. It came as a surprise to them and to everyone when they learned of this sudden, unexpected decision to retire.

An advertisement was immediately placed in the local paper announcing my retirement in two weeks. In it, patients were advised that they could pick up their records or have them sent to another doctor of their choice.

My allergy patients represented an additional difficult problem since they were dependent on me for regular injections at one-, two-, or three-week intervals. I was determined that no one would have his or her course of treatment interrupted or discontinued because I was no longer available. This meant that in two weeks' time, it would be necessary to give them their final injection in my office and provide them with an extract (their specific allergy medicine for injection) to take to another doctor to continue the treatment. The medications were so specific that no one else could provide them for my patients.

Since I had no nurse, it meant that I had to give all the injections and prepare all the extracts myself with the help of someone to assist me. This is time consuming, requiring careful attention to sterility and accuracy without being interrupted. During the day, there was no time to do this properly.

In this emergency, these preparations had to be done at night and weekends, and my regular employees couldn't be there. Fortunately, a bright but untrained family friend was unemployed. She agreed to work temporarily to help me prepare the extracts. During the two weeks, every patient's medication and schedule of injections was prepared. It was hard work, but when completed, my anxiety regarding these patients was alleviated. Another load was lifted from my shoulders.

My secretaries had to cancel all appointments that had previously been scheduled beyond the closing date and try to help patients find other doctors. Before my secretary was to leave, she tried her best to bring all billings and insurance forms that had to be completed up to date. There was too much to be done in this short time, and many tasks were left for completion after the closing date.

It was with a heavy heart that I faced each day leading to my retirement, but there was also much consolation from the outpouring of thanks, laudatory expressions, and good wishes from patients and my many co-workers and associates who had been part of my life for many years.

Chapter 3

Near the end of April 1980, I saw my last patient and ended my involvement in the active practice of medicine. It was difficult emotionally but also a relief. Now it would be possible to rest my eyes and determine how much recovery from the double vision could occur spontaneously. The last month had been very stressful trying to work as an impaired physician without adequate office help, especially since the workload for everyone was heavier than usual.

Under normal circumstances, I would not accompany my wife to her conference, which was to start soon. We decided that since I was now retired, the first and best way to take advantage of my freedom would be to go on a mini vacation by joining her at the conference. Getting away from home and relaxing in the comfortable hotel without any demands on me turned out to be a very good move. It was most enjoyable watching how capably my wife conducted the meetings and listening to her excellent speeches and delivery.

It was her big moment, and I basked in her reflected glory. Although I had to repeatedly relate what had happened to me to my many friends there, it didn't bother me.

Disengagement from a lifetime career can be difficult, but here, it started smoothly with my thoughts on things other than my problems. I was having a good time with nothing to do but eat, sleep, socialize, and relax. This was great for me, but I would be going home soon to face reality. I was getting ready to meet the challenges that lay ahead.

What were these challenges? My life was in crisis. No longer did I enjoy the status, the professional satisfactions, enjoyment, and income of a fulfilling career. Now that my life was so disrupted, trying to flagellate myself for not having more foresight would serve no useful purpose.

Although I had suffered from severe hyperthyroidism the year before, my recovery seemed complete and my health good. Practicing solo rather than with a partner had always been my preference. My colleagues in our specialty were all compatible, and we had an efficient coverage arrangement to take time off. With no children at home, my wife and I were able to take vacations and travel as we pleased. Life seemed good, so why worry?

Retirement was not a priority in the "golden age of medicine." This is an apt description of the years following World War II when my medical cohorts and I entered and practiced medicine. It was a time of spectacular technological advances which enabled us to bring previously undreamed-of help to our patients. Physicians were held in high esteem as our practices flourished in a time of continued prosperity.

A majority of our patients had health insurance with few restrictions. Most policies paid for hospital workups but not for outpatient diagnostic studies. Therefore, patients demanded and expected to be hospitalized for these studies even when it was unnecessary. There was no outpatient surgery, and even minor operations were done in the main operating rooms following which the patients went home. There was no motivation to do minor procedures in a doctor's office as long as insurance paid the bill.

Although there was overuse of insurance, patients were generally pleased and satisfied with their doctors and the attention they received. Professional life for physicians could be carried on without the stress of quarreling with insurance companies that were denying their patients appropriate care that was to occur in more recent times. Hospitals and physicians prospered. It was a wonderful time to be in the practice of medicine because of the feeling that everything you wanted to do to benefit your patient could be done without interference from third parties.

Medicine is a demanding profession, but in this golden age, it was also very enjoyable and very satisfying. The last thing most of us were thinking about was retirement. I did not plan for it except perhaps when my golf game was so awful. When tempted to quit playing golf because of my frustration, I did jokingly say, "Perhaps someday I will retire and have time on my hands. If I quit now, I may well be very sorry in the future."

Thoughts about financing retirement were forced on physicians rather than sought when organized medicine was dragged screaming into the Social Security System. Later on, when Keough Plans and IRAs became available, I took advantage of them.

Then the unexpected happened. My unanticipated forced retirement was traumatic and devastating. I was totally unprepared for the future. My status and professional income disappeared overnight.

I felt that my life was over, but fortunately, it was only temporarily on hold. This is the story of a new beginning. Since every new beginning must start with an ending, it is necessary to familiarize you with the first sixty-six years of my life that had come to a halt.

Chapter 4

In the following story, there is a one-sentence summary of my life up to this point. Many years ago, my wife and I were honored at a dinner by one of our chosen charities for our hard work and contributions in its behalf. As often happens, the program was running very late, and everyone was tired and anxious to have it end. The award had been made to us. We both were prepared to give an appropriate response, but because of the late hour, my wife whispered to me that I alone should respond and get it over fast.

To digress for a moment, it has always been one of my mental exercises to develop abstract ideas that I could store away for future stories, jokes, or writings. One such idea was to very briefly summarize my life and what had influenced it. This had been thought out and stored in my mind.

Instead of using my prepared remarks, the following rolled off my lips, "Thank you for the honor you have bestowed on us this evening. If I am deserving of this honor, it is for the following three reasons: First, I chose my parents very carefully; second, I made a very wise choice of a wife; and third, because I think God gave me enough sense not to spit in my own well. Thank you very much." Probably no one was listening, but there was the usual round of applause. The evening was over.

To elaborate on this, my carefully chosen parents were Mary and Charles Friedman who, as teenagers, had arrived in America from Eastern Europe through Ellis Island in the early 1900s. Mary was a born storyteller whose description of the horrors of her boat trip in steerage to these shores as well as the hardships my father suffered getting here left an indelible impression on me of the greatness of America.

My father was a tailor, and my mother worked as a seamstress in the garment industry in New York City. Like so many new immigrants, they lived with relatives on the Lower East Side, went to night school to learn English, and worked at their trade.

They met and became engaged, but making a living to support a family in the city was difficult. When my father was offered a good-paying opportunity as a tailor in Glens Falls, New York, two hundred miles from New York City, he grabbed it hoping he could influence his fiancée to marry him and move there—leaving several sisters, one brother and other family who provided security in this strange land and moving to the countryside where she knew no one.

My father's new boss, Pete Levitt, soon realized he was a master tailor and didn't want to lose him, which would surely happen if his bride-to-be did not want to live in the country.

Mary Haberman's first visit here was in the winter, arriving by train at Fort Edward about five miles from Glens Falls. His boss sent my father to the train station to meet her on his fancy sleigh with prancing horses, bells, and beautiful blankets. This romantic ride, her correct evaluation of the opportunity for the future, and my mother's adventuresome nature led her to say yes. My parents were married in New York City in 1910 and began their life together in this prosperous, very attractive small city in the foothills of the Adirondack Mountains. The industries were insurance, lumbering, and paper mills.

It is interesting to note that almost ninety years after our parents moved to Glens Falls, my sister who lives in Florida visited an audiologist to obtain a hearing aid. In a discussion, it turned out that the audiologist was the granddaughter of my father's first boss in Glens Falls. The mother of the audiologist had been our schoolmate.

To me, it has always seemed like a blessing that my childhood was spent here. This area abounded with lakes. Further north, the mighty Hudson River arose and passed through our city where the spectacular falls gave our city its name. This great river played a vital role in the industry and history of our area.

We lived in the West End section of the city along with most of the Eastern European Jews who had come to this country in the 1880s and early 1900s. Our lifestyle had been modified for life in America, but many of the old country customs persisted. Most of the men earned a living as peddlers, junk dealers, small storekeepers, or tailors.

The neighborhood was full of children, and there was always a gang of us figuring out our own ways to keep entertained. We reported in for meals, but when we were not in school, our mothers usually didn't know where we were or what we were doing in the streets and fields around us. There were lots of wide open spaces, and we were quite creative in setting up games and finding ways to spend our time.

One of the craziest was a time when we were building cabins; actually they were shallow underground caves. We must have been pretty good engineers because they never collapsed on us. After the cave was completed, we would sit around telling stories and trying to smoke cigarettes made out of corn silk. However, this lacked real excitement until someone suggested that we fill the cave with brush, light the brush, and have a contest to see who could stay in the smoke-filled area the longest. We did just that. Although it was dangerous, no one was hurt. I remember getting out pretty fast and definitely was not the winner.

My early years are full of stories, four of which were published in the book *Hometown Memories: Recollections of Glens Falls in the 40s, 30s and Before*, pages 20 to 24, published in October 2000.

Hometown Memories II, which was published in October 2002, contains an article by me on pages 19 to 26 about the West End section of Glens Falls during my youth. The name of the publisher does not appear in either of the two books.

Chapter 5

I was the middle child in our family. My sister Martha is twenty-one months older, and my brother Moe is seven years younger than I. We were always a close-knit family and have remained so to this day.

Those Jews living in the West End belonged to the Orthodox synagogue, the only one until 1925, when a Reform temple was built. I went to Hebrew school after school where I learned to read Hebrew but nothing about our rich history, culture, and traditions. Most of what was done from a religious standpoint was done blindly out of faith or superstition because that was the only approach our parents and teachers knew. That was the norm for the time, and my religious education would have probably been as deficient no matter where we lived.

In those days, if you wanted to learn to play a musical instrument like the violin, by your successful completion of a course of lessons, you were given the violin by the teacher. My parents made me start on such a course, but after a few lessons, the teacher told my parents I could never learn to play and not waste the money on me. That was when they learned I was tone deaf and had no appreciation for music. It was fine with me that I did not have to practice and try to play the violin.

Most of our spare time at home was spent reading, and we became voracious readers. Those of us in the neighborhood who were myopic (nearsighted) started to wear glasses at an early age. It was rumored that we had to wear glasses because we ruined our eyes reading too much in poor light. Becoming a bookworm at an early age with a love for reading has greatly enriched my life.

My mother was an attractive woman and an excellent actress. In my very early years, there was an amateur Yiddish theater group in our area, and my mother always played the lead as well as singing and dancing. My father was the stage manager and played minor parts. Even my sister was drafted when a child was needed. Rehearsals were often held in our home, and some of my fondest memories go back to these exciting evenings. The night the play was presented was the big social and cultural event of the year for our community.

This influenced my interest in theater in high school and college where I was a member of casts in minor roles.

About the time I was born, my father left his employer and established his own tailoring business and, later, a men's store. Saturday was the big business day, and he worked on Saturday in order to make a living. My mother helped him in the store on Saturdays, and they had to find something for me to do. They gave me a quarter for the afternoon. This paid for two hot dogs and a bottle of soda for lunch (fifteen cents), five cents for the movies and five cents for candies. The Park Theater was always full of kids on Saturday afternoon, watching the exciting silent movies.

In the early 1920s, when I was eight years old, my parents opened a summer business in Schroon Lake, a popular summer resort town about forty miles north of Glens Falls. This move resulted in a change in our family lifestyle. Spending summers there in my formative years led to experiences that helped shape my development. A beautiful beach was nearby, and we had to go there to swim without any parental supervision. We were careful and behaved. We also were introduced to fishing.

When I was a little older, I began to caddy on the golf links. It meant getting up very early in the morning to get in line because you were assigned to a player by your position in the line of caddies. Competition was fierce, and some older boys from out of town even camped nearby to be first. We called them "the bandits."

If you were lucky, you could carry two bags in the morning for eighteen holes, eat your brown-bag lunch, and then do the same thing in the afternoon. It was hard work walking thirty-six holes, many of them hilly, in the hot sun. With tips, you could earn $5 a day, which was quite a lot of money in the 1920s.

However, to add to my education, there was a crap game every day late in the afternoon which attracted me. Sometimes I won, and other times I lost. I never can forget the look on my mother's face when I returned home exhausted and without any money after working from early morning. She didn't say much, but I was learning the hard way the truth of the expression I have used with my children, "A fool and his money are soon parted." As a result, although I have gambled, it has been mostly very conservatively and not an important part of my life.

The benefit of being introduced to golf at an early age and starting to play then resulted in a hobby that has been important in my life. I lacked natural athletic ability and never became a good golfer.

It didn't take long before my father gave up his business in Glens Falls, and he and my mother concentrated on the summer business. As my sister and I grew older, we began to work in the store so my father could spend more time tailoring, which he loved and did so well. It was truly a family business and one of the great learning experiences of our young lives.

We learned by example from our parents the meaning of hard work and cooperation. Our philosophy, as enunciated by our mother, was, "If we all work together, we will all have something; if we don't, no one will have anything." We developed a work ethic along with salesmanship, an understanding of interpersonal relationships, the value of honesty, reliability, control of one's emotions under difficult circumstances, and fair dealing. I have been forever grateful to my parents for the lifestyle and lessons learned from them that helped me develop into a mature and self-reliant person at an early age.

Just to show how much was learned by example, the following observation made a tremendous impression on my youthful mind. At the time, there was no bank in town. My father was good at handling money, and customers trusted him. One of the town alcoholics had earned over $500 (a lot of money in the 1920s) and had it in cash. It was Friday, and he knew he would blow the money over the weekend. He said to my father, "Charlie, hold this for me over the weekend." He handed my father $500 in cash, didn't ask for a receipt, and said, "I'll see you Monday," as he walked out. On Monday, he showed up, collected his money and said, "Thanks." Incidents like this were repeated again and again and established my determination to be as respected and trustworthy as my father.

The use of "common sense" was emphasized by our parents, who related it to good judgement. It was not something that could be taught. They often used the term "educated fools" when referring to people who had good formal educations but did not get anywhere because they lacked common sense.

With the passing years, my loving remembrance and appreciation of my parents increases more and more.

Chapter 6

Not much mention has been made of my brother, Moey Leo Friedman, who was seven years younger than I. It was my responsibility to take him to the beach, but I don't recall spending much time with him except at meals.

At an early age, he caddied on the golf links, and he loved fishing. While still too young to work in our store, he started a bait business in the store basement, which eventually developed into quite an operation with considerable equipment, the centerpiece of which was an old bathtub with running water.

His stock consisted of worms (nightcrawlers), minnows, frogs, crawfish, and other bait. Since he couldn't be there all the time, if, in his absence, a bait customer came into the store for worms, rather than lose a sale, one of us who was there would go down in the basement and get them. My sister Martha hated worms, but she had a special pair of gloves to wear when handling them. Most of the other types of bait were left to him to dispense.

We must have appeared a little strange with these goings-on, and there were some zany happenings like the famous Friedman frog hunt which occurred at a time when I was not home.

Moe was expecting a shipment of frogs one day, and the supplier didn't deliver them until late at night when the store was closed and our parents were asleep in our apartment above the store. Rather than awaken my father for the keys to open the store, he decided to keep the frogs in water in the deep part of our double kitchen sink. It had a cover which he left slightly open to provide air, never thinking the frogs could get out.

My father was always the first one up in the morning and was shocked to see frogs on the bed, under the bed, and all over the house. Everyone was awakened and began catching the jumping, elusive frogs. The hunt took an exciting and frustrating two hours before things were back to normal. When Moe tells the story, in retrospect, it seems so funny he can't control his laughter.

During those years, our family led a dual existence. During the school months, we lived in Glens Falls and had what might be called a normal life. In the summer months, our personal lives were on hold while we worked in our store twelve to fourteen hours a day for six days. On Sundays, we closed early so we could go to the movies or just rest. Despite the hardships, we found pleasure and humor in our work. At the end of the season for the Jewish holidays, we would go to the famous Scaroon Manor Hotel. This was our main family vacation together.

In 1929, my parents built a building in Schroon Lake and planned to live there instead of Glens Falls. This presented no problem for Moe who was nine years old, but Martha was going into her senior year in the Glens Falls High School. It was my junior year. All our close friends were in Glens Falls, and I was on the football team. We were devastated by the thought of moving to another school. We lived in a rented apartment and prevailed on our parents to allow just the two of us to remain in the apartment in Glens Falls and go to school there. Our parents were very understanding. Since Martha could cook, and they felt we were responsible and trustworthy, our wish was granted. We were good kids, and all went well. My sister graduated and went to New York City to work. My parents then gave up the apartment.

I was a senior and most anxious to graduate from the Glens Falls High School. Among our neighbors and friends was a family who took in boarders. One of their sons was a friend and classmate of mine. I had always spent a good deal of time in their home and was comfortable there. My understanding parents agreed to allow me to board there for the school year. It was hard for them because it was 1930 and the beginning of the Depression. I graduated with my class.

During high school, our group of male friends didn't date girls except to go to an affair like the junior prom. There were few mixed parties, and most of our activities were male oriented, such as sports.

It was understood that I was to go to college. Because of their limited formal education, my parents wanted their sons to be college educated. That meant you went to college to become something by preparing to enter a profession. My guidance counselor had told me that in seeking a career to aim high.

My first interest was in becoming an optometrist. I thought that applying to the Columbia University School of Optometry in New York City was all I had to do. Since I was naive and did not realize how severe the competition was, to my surprise and chagrin, my application was rejected.

By this time, it was early summer. My parents were not familiar with colleges and left the choice up to me. I knew someone who was a junior at Union College in Schenectady and asked him about the school. He strongly recommended it, and I applied and was accepted. There optometry was no longer an option, and since I had to be something, I decided to take a premedical course.

Union College was all-male and a fraternity-dominated school at that time with very limited dormitory space. Freshmen were sought after by the fraternities in advance of their arrival on the campus and moved right into the houses as pledges when college started. My friend belonged to Kappa Nu Fraternity and steered me there. I found fraternity life very much to my liking and lived in the fraternity house for all four years.

We had an alumnus adviser who lived in Schenectady and helped the elected student officers with the management of the fraternity house—its finances, the dining facilities, and the employees. One of the students was the steward, who collected the rent, acted as liaison with the employees, and paid the bills. After having been there only a few weeks as a pledge, our adviser approached me and asked me to serve as the steward. It was obvious no one wanted the job (money was scarce, and there were no benefits). It was flattering to think that as a pledge, they considered me capable enough to take on this responsibility. My answer was yes.

Being steward entailed collecting room and board, and most of the members paid regularly. However, there was a sophomore who was the only real playboy among us. His family had been wealthy, but the Depression had hit them hard. They cut their son's allowance considerably, and instead of paying his obligations to us, he spent it on his dates. He was in arrears, and I kept bugging him to pay up to no avail. The fraternity was just getting by financially, so I warned him I would contact his father and inform him of his son's debt. This member ignored me, and I did write the letter which explained the problem. I asked that his room and board checks be sent directly to me.

The father never contacted me, but the culprit threatened to beat me up if I ever wrote to his father again. However, I had no problem collecting from him after that, and we remained friendly.

Chapter 7

For me, fraternity life was an excellent social and living arrangement. Most of the freshmen in our house came to college with good scholastic records and limited social experience. The fraternity provided compatible companionship and friendships that lasted long after graduation. When there were dances, the upperclassmen found dates for us. After Prohibition was repealed, there was moderate drinking. Smoking cigarettes was popular. Bull sessions, usually about girls and sex, were held frequently. We were mostly talk.

The premedical course was arduous. Knowing how difficult it was to get into medical school, especially for a Jew, motivated me to work very hard at my studies. Emphasis on the sciences precluded taking desirable courses in the humanities. A course in chemistry called Quantitative Analysis was scary because everything depended on one chance to do an experiment correctly. If you failed that course, you might well forget about getting into medical school. There was a lot of pressure, but it was a good life.

Just as soon as school was out in June, my destination was Schroon Lake, to work in the family summer business. It was a perfect arrangement because this was when I was needed. In return, my parents were able to pay my college expenses.

In my senior year, I applied to many medical schools. It was a tense time because in the previous years, we had watched some students get into schools and others fail. Some had gone to schools abroad. Things looked bleak for me until the early spring when, in one unforgettable week, I was informed of my election to the Phi Beta Kappa Society and admission to the Albany Medical College.

With my career hopes on course, entering medical school in 1935 was a challenge that was faced with trepidation. We had heard horror stories about how there were not enough places in the second-year laboratories (labs) for all the entering freshmen, so a certain number would have to be flunked out. Also, because of the pressure, students worked so hard that several had developed pulmonary tuberculosis, forcing them to leave school.

However, on our first day, we received the good news that the class was smaller than in the past, with room in the second-year labs for everyone whose record was satisfactory. No one had to be flunked out. It was a great relief. We started right away in the anatomy lab dissecting the cadavers, and in the first week, two students decided they didn't want to become doctors and dropped out. To me, this was very upsetting, since there were many capable aspirants whose applications had been rejected and would have succeeded if given a chance.

The first two years of medical school were spent in labs and preclinical courses with very little exposure to patients. There was so much to learn that most of us did little but study. If there were any personal problems, you kept them to yourself. There was no counseling or coddling. Medicine was considered a very demanding profession. In preparation, you had to learn to handle all kinds of stress and fatigue in school, internship, and residency without complaining.

The final two years were spent on the wards taking care of patients. We began to feel like doctors. I'll never forget the first patient assigned to me on my first day. She was an aging lady on the medical ward with many problems. With an instructive outline to guide me, I did such a complete history and physical examination that the attention gave her the impression I knew what I was doing. She was very pleased with me.

That evening, the chief medical resident, the top man in the hierarchy, was making rounds (means visiting the patients) with his staff. They determined that the woman needed to have some minor surgery performed to improve her condition. She replied, "You can't do anything until my doctor, Dr. Friedman, gives his OK." The resident didn't even know me, and according to the story, he exploded, "Who the hell is Dr. Friedman?" Someone explained to him and the patient that I was a third-year medical student.

She accepted the explanation and acceded to their recommendation. I showed up at her bedside early the next morning, and she let me know that she knew my status. She liked my attention, was friendly, and allowed me to keep her as a patient.

After my second year, part of the summer was spent working for the last time in our store, and the rest was spent in the Albany Hospital, fulfilling my student requirements on the Obstetrical Service. After my third year, I spent the summer as a surgical extern (a student doing the work of an intern) in the hospital.

When it came time in my senior year to decide on a hospital for my one-year internship, my choice was to apply to the Beth El Hospital in Brooklyn. I wanted to be exposed to a big-city medical atmosphere after spending my previous four years in a smaller city, Albany. Beth El was a moderate-sized community hospital with much sought-after internships. However, my uncle had been president of the hospital board of directors, and he assured me of acceptance if my medical-school record and recommendations were satisfactory. I was accepted.

In later discussions with my fellow interns, I found out that almost everyone who was accepted had a connection. The way we put it was, "Who's your rabbi?" Most of the interns intended to practice in Brooklyn, and an internship in a private hospital usually assured you of a staff appointment, which was very desirable.

It was 1939, and the country still had not recovered from the Depression. Many people felt capitalism had failed and perhaps communism was the answer. My life in school had been quite sheltered. The first thing I noted in the interns' quarters was two newspapers, *The New York Times* and *The Daily Worker* (the Communist Party newspaper). Coming to New York City was an excellent move since my exposure to new and different attitudes and approaches to medical and personal situations widened my horizons as a person and doctor.

I always looked young for my age, and a ward patient of mine asked me, "Sonny, are you really a doctor?" My mother had urged me to grow a mustache because she had a premonition this would happen. I didn't like mustaches and never did grow one. The patient was reassured regarding my qualifications.

Our hospital was located on the border of Brownsville and East New York, a poor, tough area that spawned the famous gang Murder, Inc. My rotation included riding the ambulance (serving as the ambulance doctor) in this area for one month. Our instructions were to wait for a police presence before entering a home or building. Probably much more was learned about life than medicine on the ambulance. It was worthwhile.

Usually, people with injuries like lacerations were brought to the emergency room for suturing by the intern on duty there. Being "gung ho," I decided this was a waste of resources since the ambulance kit contained all the necessary supplies. It didn't take long before the call came to the home of a man whose forearm had been slashed. My decision was to suture the laceration in his home.

It turned out to be a deeper and more extensive wound than anticipated and took quite a while to sew up. The room was hot and humid. I was perspiring profusely and getting a little nervous because the room was full of family and friends crowding around me to see the operation. All ended well, as did the noble experiment of trying to be a hero.

During that year, I began to worry about a slight hearing loss that was noticeable to me but was not obvious. Since my father had developed a severe hearing loss in his middle years, this probably would happen to me. This aroused my interest in the field of otolaryngology (ear, nose, and throat). Also, the use of a stethoscope would not be crucial as in a medical specialty. It was necessary to make a career choice to follow my internship. For me, it was ear, nose, and throat if I could get admitted to a training program, which was very difficult and competitive.

Chapter 8

In 1939, a medical-school graduate usually served a one-year hospital internship during which it was customary to spend a month at a time working in a different specialized field. It was called a rotating internship. If a doctor wanted to enter general practice, he or she could do so after this one year.

To specialize in a particular field like medicine, pediatrics, obstetrics, surgery, or ear, nose, and throat, the doctor spent a couple of years or more gaining further training as a hospital resident gaining extensive experience in the chosen specialty.

The number of aspirants seeking specialization was usually much greater than the available desirable residencies, and competition was fierce for these positions. Another track that had recently developed was to take a basic science and introductory course as a student physician in a university setting. After such a one-year course, it was easier to get a residency. Also, this could replace the first year of residency. These programs were expensive and much sought after.

By this time, I was twenty-six years old and still dependent on my parents, since, as an intern, I received room, board, and laundry but no salary. My loving parents had generously provided for me, but they had warned me about marriage saying, "We can support one but not two." This presented no problem since my future was so unsettled that marriage was not on my mind. At that time, the Beth El Hospital required that their interns be single. Marriage was not allowed, and if it was discovered that an intern was married, he would be fired. It was expected that your time and energy would be devoted to the hospital. We worked long hours and very hard.

The University of Pennsylvania in Philadelphia presented a highly regarded basic science course in otolaryngology. It would be an expensive year, but again, my parents said they would provide the funds if I went there. The hospital gave me excellent recommendations, and I was overjoyed to be accepted into the program which started in the fall of 1940.

My year as an intern was a learning experience which required long hours and hard work without much fresh air and sunshine. When it ended in June of 1940, I was exhausted. The summer months were free and provided an opportunity to rehabilitate myself by taking a job as a camp doctor in a summer camp for boys in the Adirondack Mountains, about fifteen miles from my home in Schroon Lake.

In those days, we did not know how harmful smoking was, and most of the doctors smoked. It was my feeling that heavy smoking contributed to my fatigue, and I resolved to quit smoking that summer and did.

Although most of my time had to be spent at the camp, the work was not hard with time to take advantage of the lake, fresh air, and sunshine. Not smoking helped, and by the end of the summer, my energy and sense of well-being had been regained.

Being a camp doctor provided a valuable new experience for me. For the first time, I was on my own without support from teachers and colleagues in medical school and the hospital. My training had prepared me for this new level of responsibility, and fortunately, the campers and counselors were a healthy group. The biggest problem was with the owner of the camp, because after many years of experience, he felt he knew more about medical care than the newly graduated interns who worked for him. Especially sticky was deciding whether a camper was healthy enough to benefit from the program, since sending him home meant a loss of tuition.

As an example, there was a boy with severe asthma who was spending most of his time in the infirmary. I suggested to the owner that the proper approach was to send him home. There he would be in a more suitable environment where he could get adequate treatment. The owner ignored my suggestion, and the patient continued to spend most of his time in the infirmary. After four weeks of camp, there was the Parents' Weekend, and I told this boy's parents that I felt their son was not benefiting from camp because of his illness. They decided to take him home, and my boss was very angry at me, but he could not do anything about it.

We had two counselors in our camp who were football stars at a leading Ivy League college, and one was the quarterback. He injured his ankle, which looked like an ordinary sprain. I was afraid if my diagnosis was incorrect and the injury more serious and not treated properly; it might ruin his athletic career. The owner felt it was not necessary for me to take him almost fifty miles for an x-ray, but I insisted. The x-ray showed no fracture, and his ankle healed well.

Having convictions and the courage to act on my convictions was the only way I could act professionally and conduct my life.

In the fall, I enrolled as a student physician at the Graduate School of Medicine of the University of Pennsylvania. This was a comprehensive program dealing with the basic sciences in ear, nose, and throat, which are only dealt with superficially in medical school and are the foundation for practicing the specialty. We worked in clinics with patients and observed surgery.

Philadelphia was famous as the leading center in the world for laryngology and bronchoesophagology (the examination and treatment of diseases of the voice box, the bronchial tubes of the lungs, and the swallowing tube from the throat to and including the stomach). Dr. Chevalier Jackson at Temple Hospital was world famous for his innovative work in this new field, especially the removal of foreign bodies, like food, bones, and pins, from these tubes using rigid metal scopes and delicate forceps which he designed.

Aspiration of these foreign bodies usually ended in chronic illness and/or death before the introduction of these new techniques which were also used for the diagnosis and treatment of cancer and other diseases of the air and food passages. One of our professors, Dr. Gabriel Tucker, was trained by Dr. Jackson and was an expert in this field. In our program, we observed these procedures being carried out on patients and practiced them on anesthetized dogs. This was a valuable introduction to this exciting and important branch of medicine, which was one of my favorites throughout my career.

Dr. Jackson had retired, but he still lived in the area. We wanted to meet this famous physician, and our professor arranged for him to give us a guest lecture. He was an artist and illustrated his excellent presentation by making drawings on black paper with colored crayons using both hands. He made two such drawings and gave them to the class. We drew lots for them, and I won one, which I had framed and is a prized possession hanging over my desk to this day. Meeting him was a rare and enjoyable experience.

My living quarters were in the famous Rittenhouse Square in a room rented from a widow in what had been a lovely private home before the Depression took its toll. It was near the Graduate Hospital where we spent most of our time. It was also near a pharmacy which had a lunch counter where I sometimes ate. My future wife worked as a laboratory technician in the same area at that time and also ate at this lunch counter, but we never met.

The school year spent in Philadelphia was a productive learning experience. In the clinics, many of the instructors were retired specialists who gave us the benefit of their wisdom and many years of practical experience. I developed friendships with my classmates and one of the teachers that continued for many years. My training in my chosen field was launched, but the next step was to obtain a residency in a hospital for further training.

Chapter 9

In seeking a residency program in otolaryngology (ear, nose, and throat), I recalled that they had recently started a two-year program in my field at the Albany Hospital for one resident. This was the university hospital for my medical school.

The present resident would graduate on June 30, 1941. There would be a position open beginning July 1, which would be the perfect time for me to start.

As soon as I was settled in at the University of Pennsylvania (U of P), I contacted the professor who was in charge of the department at Albany about applying for the residency position. He was delighted to have an alumnus with a basic course from the U of P apply for his program and assured me I had an excellent chance of being accepted. When the appointments were made at a later time, I received it.

On July 1, 1941, I was back at the Albany Hospital among old friends and teachers after an absence of two years of a learning experience in institutions in large metropolitan areas. Seeing how medicine was practiced elsewhere definitely had broadened my understanding and perspective of how to be a good doctor.

Now, practical training in the medical and surgical aspects of my specialty under the supervision of my teachers was underway. As a resident, there was much more status and responsibility than in my past experience. My duties included conducting the outpatient clinics, assisting at surgery and performing surgery under supervision, providing preoperative and postoperative care, doing consultations and treatments on patients in other hospital services and in the emergency room.

At twenty-seven years of age, my salary was $25 a month, plus room, board, and laundry. To become a doctor meant delayed gratification regarding one's personal life. Fortunately, my parents' support had kept me out of debt.

In the ear, nose, and throat (otolaryngology) field, we dealt with medical and surgical problems of the ears, such as deafness, ear and mastoid (behind the ear) infections, and disturbances in balance (dizziness). However, since the advent of sulfa drugs, acute mastoiditis, which had been very prevalent, serious, and requiring mastoid surgery, had become quite rare.

Also included was the medical and surgical treatment of the mouth and throat (especially tonsillectomy and adenoidectomy), the larynx, the nose and sinuses, and the air and food passages.

The training of a doctor is a gradual process, and while, on a daily basis, the changes are not noticed, the accumulative effect of hard work, study, and dedication over time results in diagnostic acumen, technical skills, and the ability to carry out the appropriate treatment. This parable will illustrate what happens: "Amazingly, a farmer was able to lift up a full-grown cow. When asked how he could do this, he replied that from the day it was a little calf, he picked it up daily. From day to day, he could not discern the small increase in the animal's weight until he was lifting the full-grown cow."

In the same way, knowledge and experience increase incrementally, until you have a well-trained but still fledgling doctor. However, very important innate traits such as empathy, viewing the patient as a person and not a case, along with the ability to communicate, are not and usually cannot be taught in any training program. Either you have them or you don't.

In medical school, I had passed the National Board examinations and, by this time, was licensed to practice medicine and surgery in New York State.

The morning of December 7, 1941 (the day that President Roosevelt said, "Would live in infamy,") is indelibly imprinted in my mind. I was seeing a patient in the emergency room (ER) when the news of the attack on Pearl Harbor spread through the ER like wildfire. Everyone was shocked. Little did I realize at that moment how this event would change my plans and my life.

With the declaration of war against Japan and Germany following Pearl Harbor, there was a rapid buildup of our armed forces, and doctors were in great demand. I was single, in my second year of specialty training, and, therefore, subject to be drafted. The rumor was if you volunteered, you would get a better assignment, so I volunteered to serve after completing my year as a resident in June 1942.

Although it was with regret that I had to forego the second year of residency training, my experience qualified me as a specialist, and the army promised to recognize me as an otolaryngologist and assign me in my chosen field. Considering that many of my future military professional colleagues would be required to leave established lifestyles with homes, families, and practices, my situation was really quite good.

The army physical examination was passed without difficulty, and because of my slight hearing loss, they placed me on "limited service," which theoretically would keep me out of a combat zone. I was given a commission as a first lieutenant in the Medical Corps of the Army of the United States. This was to distinguish us newcomers from the regular (or professional) army called the United States Army, which never really accepted us as their equals in the military.

Being a close-knit family made it especially painful for my parents, family, as well as friends to see me leave them and go to war. It was easier for me since, for many years, my life had been spent away from home. Besides my immediate family ties, I had no attachments or responsibility to anyone that I was being wrenched away from. My outlook was that of adventure of the unknown and a new experience. Professionally, I expected to work in my field. Being an officer brought status and a salary that would make me self-supporting for the first time in my life.

My residency ended on June 30. After three weeks of vacation at home, with lumps in all our throats, I said goodbye to my family in July 1942 and took the train to my first assignment in Camp Lee, Virginia.

Chapter 10

Camp Lee was located in Petersburg, Virginia, near Richmond and was a very large quartermaster training base. The Quartermaster Corps is the army department that provides clothing and subsistence for a body of troops. Thousands of new recruits came directly there from induction centers for basic training.

An officer candidate school (OCS) for quartermasters was also located there. Enlisted men chosen for officer's training went through three months of rigorous training and were graduated as officers, second lieutenants, the so-called ninety-day wonders.

If my recall is correct, there were about forty thousand soldiers on the base. Petersburg was famous for the Crater, a large bomb crater from Civil War days which was a historical site.

I was immediately assigned to the eye, ear, nose, and throat department and underwent no orientation or basic training beforehand. Later on, there was some training like the firing range and going through the obstacle course where we crawled on our bellies with live ammunition being fired over our heads. There was a shortage of doctors in our department, and my professional colleagues were delighted to see me and put me to work right away.

Every new recruit had to be examined by our department as part of a comprehensive examination, and for hours, my duty was to do routine ear, nose, and throat (ENT) examinations of one person after another, which can be quite boring. The rough afternoons occurred after all the enlisted men had hamburgers and onions for lunch and then repeatedly breathed the strong smell of onion in my face when asked to say "Ah," with a tongue depressor pressing on their tongues.

One of the bonuses was to look at a recruit and recognize a friend or acquaintance from the past. There was time for only a very brief chat that ended because the line had to keep moving. Unhappily for me, because of the army rule that officers and enlisted men did not fraternize, I was unable to follow up on these contacts and meet at a later time. This resulted from a lesson that was learned shortly after coming to Camp Lee when an enlisted man, a close friend and college fraternity brother, Milton Schwebel, and I tried to meet. There was no place where we could be comfortably be seen together or even sit down, relax, and talk.

Because of the segregation required by military discipline, artificially, my position was that of his superior. It was a discomforting experience, especially since he was my equal or more intellectually and in ability. Rather than having enjoyed myself, the meeting left me tense from guilt feelings and anger at the system.

Some disorders were found among the recruits that would require treatment or surgery or even discharge from the service. The local draft boards were so anxious to fill their quotas that they inducted men with problems like very severe deafness knowing full well they were unfit for military duty and would be rejected before basic training began.

My other duties included conducting clinics and performing some surgery. All the new recruits who needed them were fitted with eyeglasses that had to be ordered from a laboratory by requisition. All five copies of each requisition had to be signed individually (no carbon copies allowed) by an officer. Although my duties did not include eye work, as a member of the department, I had to take my turn at signing my name on hundreds of orders daily. This was my introduction to boring army paperwork.

Virginia was farther south than I had ever been, and the summer weather was brutally hot and humid. Our quarters were wooden one-story buildings with tin roofs. They were as comfortable as a Turkish bath. The best you could do in the evening trying to be comfortable was lie on your bunk and just sweat.

In many ways, army living for an officer was not much different from living in hospital quarters to which I was accustomed. We had single rooms, shared bathrooms, card and sitting rooms. Our meals were taken in the officers' mess hall (dining room) and were served cafeteria style. For one accustomed to institutional food, there was variety and a good menu. Having been brought up not to waste food, the army motto "Take all you can eat, eat all you take" impressed me.

It was not difficult making friends with my medical and dental colleagues and the nurses in our unit. The Saturday night dances at the Officers Club were the big social event of the week and much enjoyed. Drinking was a part of the life, although for me it was in moderation, and before long, I started smoking again and was back to a package of cigarettes daily. The harmful effects of smoking were still unknown then, and the best gift was to give soldiers cigarettes. For a single officer, it was a pretty good life.

The transition to military life would appear on the surface as a continuation of the changes from college to medical school to internship, specialization, and residency. However, in those days, all these previous transitions were in the direction of a generally accepted goal, which was to become a doctor and establish a practice. Hopefully, the delayed gratification regarding marriage, family, and community life would be over.

The war had changed everything. The comfortable direction of my life and that of millions of other Americans had been altered. Where an orderly future had appeared almost in my grasp, there was now complete uncertainty about what lay ahead. These questions came into mind: how long will this last? where in the world would I be sent? would I become ill, wounded, incapacitated or die? would we win the war? and what kind of world would we be living in, win or lose? would I ever see my family and friends again? would there be marriage, a family, or a career in my future? Since there were no immediate answers and there was little one could do to influence the course of events, the best approach was just to live from day to day without being too contemplative.

It was getting to be a comfortable way of life by the fall of 1943, and after two hot summers in Virginia, a few colleagues who were friendly talked about renting a camp on the James River nearby for a fun time the next summer.

Also that fall, I became friendly with one of the nurses in our unit which resulted in a meaningful but strange relationship. We were attracted to each other, but she would not go out with me. Because I was quite persistent and she developed some trust in me, she eventually told me she was engaged to a soldier who had just started the Officer Candidate School for three months. She saw him on weekends, but the weeks were long and lonely. We were very comfortable with each other and found a great deal to talk about beyond the superficial level of most relationships in our milieu.

She told me she would go out with me during the week providing there would be no intimacy whatsoever between us. I was ready to agree to anything just to be with her, and we kept the bargain throughout the few months together. We found we could talk frankly to each other about our lives, the frustrations and changes caused by the war, our uncertainty and hopes for the future. Talking about our pent-up feelings somehow eased the nagging emotional pain of our lives. We both wrote poetry, and one evening, after watching the sunset, this poem developed in my mind, and I recited it out loud.

The night was dark, serene, and calm,
Just like a surgeon's healing balm,
To place upon a weary soul,
And make a broken spirit whole.

Somehow, I always felt that these few words expressed our personal struggles and the solace we felt by being together.

If this was falling in love, it was a somewhat new and bittersweet experience. While having fun, the knowledge that the relationship would soon be over saved me the agony of considering whether to marry a woman of a different faith. In the 1940s, intermarriage was not accepted as it is today, and for me to marry a woman who was not Jewish would be a terrible blow to my parents and family who had been so loving and supportive over the years. Because of my love and gratitude towards my parents and my inability to hurt them, it is most likely that my own desires and immediate happiness would have been sacrificed.

As expected, the relationship ended, and we parted good friends. I felt sad but was not devastated. Life would go on for the present without great enthusiasm.

Chapter 11

Even the ending of my relationship with my friend did not tempt me to request a transfer elsewhere to forget her (like in the old movies about joining the French Foreign Legion). After almost eighteen months in the ear, nose, and throat department at Camp Lee, I began to think of myself as so essential there that probably this would be my assignment for the rest of the war. We were always short of doctors, and replacements often were transferred elsewhere after a short stay. If they could not function without me at Camp Lee, in my mind, it meant not being transferred to an assignment overseas where life could be a horror story. Not seeking a change was acceptable to me.

However, according to army tradition, a better course would have been to ask for a transfer overseas since the military usually responded to assignment requests by giving you the opposite of what you wanted.

About this time, two soldiers under my care in the hospital presented unusually interesting and challenging medical problems. I was anxious to study the medical literature to provide the best possible care, and the camp medical library was inadequate for this study. There was an excellent medical library in Richmond where the needed references would be available. My plans were to go there on the next Saturday afternoon, but gasoline was rationed even for the military. My coupons had been used up, and my gas tank almost empty. My car could not be used.

A dentist in our unit had a girlfriend in Richmond whom he visited on Saturdays. On Friday, I asked him if it would be possible to ride with him to Richmond the next day. He was very agreeable and asked, "How would you like a date for Saturday night?" He explained his girlfriend's cousin from another city was visiting her, and we could make it a foursome. He didn't know anything about the cousin.

My mood was such that a "blind date" didn't interest me in the least, but there was no way to say no under the circumstances. Apparently, his girlfriend had asked him to find her cousin a date, and he had not done so. My request for a ride was most fortuitous for him. My reply was an obviously unenthusiastic yes.

The plan was to let me off at the library for the afternoon. Around 5 PM, I would call him at his girlfriend's home, and they would come and pick me up to go out to dinner. My research was productive, which made me feel good, but my feelings about the date were still negative.

It was dark when I was picked up and introduced to my date, Blossom Levitz, whom I joined in the backseat. Because of my unhappy mood, I spoke like a "wise guy," which was completely out of character for me. By the time we reached the restaurant, she would have gladly thrown me out of the car. Once inside and seated at our table, after a few minutes of looking at Blossom and listening to her talk, I was fascinated and had a revelation, this is my "dream girl." Now, wanting to make a good impression, I reverted to my normal self, trying to be friendly, considerate, and good company. We had an enjoyable time, and since she would be leaving in a few days to return to her home in Lebanon, Pennsylvania, I asked her for another date, and she accepted. She explained that she was attending Lebanon Valley College near her home and was having her Christmas vacation. After the second date, I told her I wanted to stay in touch and see her again. She agreed. My mood was rosy.

A few days later, orders came through for me to go on detached service (a temporary change from a regular assignment) to Camp A.P. Hill in Fredericksburg, Virginia, for about three weeks. This made me realize I wasn't an indispensable fixture at Camp Lee after all.

We lived in the field in tents in freezing January weather. There was no way to really keep warm. My assignment was as a medical officer, not as a specialist. Many of the soldiers were in the infirmary, also a tent, with colds and respiratory infections. It was my judgement that having them undress for an examination in the cold was more dangerous than leaving them alone. With rest and less exposure to the elements, most of my patients recovered quickly. It was a new experience teaching me how tough life in the field can be even when you are not fighting.

Shortly after returning to Camp Lee, orders came through transferring me to Fort Meade, Maryland, where I joined the 93rd General Hospital as the officer in charge of the ear, nose, and throat department. We knew we were going overseas.

As soon as there was a free weekend, I arranged to visit Blossom in Lebanon. After meeting her parents in her home, we were sitting around talking over coffee and cake. Her mother had baked a delicious sponge cake which was my favorite cake. She was favorably impressed by the fact that I ate several pieces and kept complimenting her on how good the cake was. They were a big family, and I was introduced to a number of family members and friends. It was a very enjoyable visit.

Sometime in March, we received our orders that we were going to the United Kingdom (England). We had a short leave, during which I had a date with Blossom in Philadelphia to say goodbye. We did a great deal of talking about our feelings for each other, but all we could do was promise to write and hope for the best under these terribly uncertain circumstances.

There was time for me to drive home to Schroon Lake to leave my car and personal belongings and say an emotional goodbye to my family. By this time, my brother was also in the army.

In March, we were transferred to Fort Dix and soon boarded the luxury liner, *The Aquitania*, which had become a troopship, and sailed out of New York Harbor past the Statue of Liberty eastward on the Atlantic Ocean where German U-boats (submarines) were known to be lurking.

Chapter 12

Traveling as an officer on a troopship was a luxury cruise compared to the hardships of the enlisted men. We shared staterooms and ate in the dining room on tables for four with tablecloths and silverware settings. The ship's regular white-jacketed waiters served us at breakfast and dinner. No lunch was served, but there was food available in the dining room to be taken to be eaten in our rooms at lunchtime.

At our table were three doctors and a chaplain. Starting with the first meal, one of the doctors and the chaplain were seasick. They hardly ate the entire trip. The other doctor and I felt good and ate everything in sight.

Time was spent walking on deck, reading, and playing cards. We were on a fast ship and had no convoy. It ran a zigzag course to avoid U-boats, which were frequently rumored to be following us.

Once, I was assigned to examine the soldiers in the hold (the bottom of the ship) where they lay in hammocks stacked one above the other. The ventilation was poor, and it was not a pleasant experience. Another day, my assignment was mess officer in the enlisted men's mess hall. It was sickening. Some of the soldiers would vomit, drop their trays, their clothes soiled, or just sitting with a glazed expression. Areas of the floor were covered with food and vomit, and the cleaning crew was kept busy. Many, however, were able to make it through the meal even under these conditions.

After about a week at sea on a clear, sunny day near the end of March 1944, our ship entered the resplendent estuary leading to the harbor in Glasgow, Scotland. From there we took a train to Colwyn Bay, Wales, a resort city on the sea. Our rooms were in summer villas with little fireplaces, but there was no wood anywhere to be found for warmth in the freezing weather. Our unit arrived before our permanent hospital site in England was ready, and there was nowhere else to send us. There was nothing for us to do. To keep busy and active, this full hospital complement of highly trained doctors, nurses, and other personnel practiced marching in formation up and down the streets.

Fortunately for me, several of us were sent on detached service to Kilrea, Northern Ireland, to run a station hospital for a couple of months. Kilrea was about twenty-five miles from Belfast where we enjoyed visiting and going to the greyhound dog races. The famous Old Bleach Linen Factory was near our town, but disappointedly, nothing could be purchased because they were making duck cloth for the military. The Old Bushmill Irish Whiskey Distillery was nearby, and we were well supplied. Of great interest for me were the fairs and markets held in the town.

At the end of this pleasant interlude, our group rejoined the 93rd General Hospital at our permanent location in Great Malvern in the Midland area of Great Britain. We were part of a general-hospital center, a cluster of hospitals designated as the highest level of military hospitals in the European Theater of Operations (the ETO), formed to care for the anticipated casualties from the invasion of the European mainland.

Our first patients from the invasion of France arrived about one week after D-day, June 6, 1944. They had been treated in field and station hospitals on the mainland before coming to us, and most of them had very serious injuries. In my department were young men with destroyed eardrums and severe or total deafness. To make it worse, some of them were also blind. There were deforming injuries to the face and sinuses. The statement "War is Hell" only begins to describe the horrible effects of war. Never before this time or after it did I ever see anything so terribly destructive to young lives.

It was the mission of our hospital to treat and rehabilitate the soldiers who could return to duty. The others were treated and stabilized and sent to military hospitals in the United States. As the war in Europe continued, so did our flow of patients.

On several occasions, I was sent to London to attend conferences, and these provided an opportunity for a little rest and recreation (R&R).

These visits gave me the chance to explore the city and its historical sites. Also seen was the destruction caused by the "buzz bombs" and life in a major city under wartime conditions, especially the sight of people sleeping in the subways for safety from the bombs. In the crowded Trafalgar Square of London, one evening, I unexpectedly met a friend, a soldier, Chester Cole, from Schroon Lake.

I kept up a correspondence with my family at home, and besides letters, they would send me food packages containing delicacies, like salami, which were shared with my buddies. In one package, the casing of the salami was broken in transit, and when opened, the stink was awful.

I wrote to Blossom frequently, often writing her poems, to which she replied. Our friendship developed in this way into a more romantic relationship. One of my standard jokes was "Because of my knack for writing, I romanced her better from a distance than in person." However, every letter from her was opened with trepidation in fear of finding it to be a "Dear John" letter, famous in the military for telling a boyfriend she was engaged to someone else and to forget her. Our common expression was "Absence makes the heart fonder for someone else." Fortunately, it didn't happen to me like to some others whom we knew.

Mail is great for the morale of soldiers, as determined by my personal experience and the information gained from the duty of censoring mail written by the enlisted men before it was sent home. The so-called purpose was to make sure no military secrets were sent in the mail where often the most intimate personal feelings were expressed. I did not like this duty.

A memorable incident occurred in September 1944 when my brother Moe arrived in England with his unit for one month there before going to France. Not knowing how to contact me, he called the Red Cross, and in ten minutes, he was talking to me on the telephone. He arranged a three-day leave to visit me, and it was wonderful getting together.

Moe was a noncommissioned officer, a sergeant. According to army protocol, he was not allowed to eat in the officers' mess hall.

When the person in charge tried to keep him out, I said firmly, "He is my brother, and he is going to eat with me here." That settled the matter, and we had all our meals together.

Because frostbite of the toes was a common injury suffered by soldiers in the field, I asked my brother about the kind of socks he had been issued and found out they would be inadequate under freezing conditions in the field. I had some real good woolen socks and gave them to him. After the war, Moe told me that many men in his outfit suffered from frostbitten toes, but my socks kept him from harm.

At the end of this morale-building visit, I promised to get a three-day leave and go see him. Before that time arrived, the Red Cross informed me my brother had left. Probably when they received orders to move, no outside calls could be made to avoid giving away any kind of information helpful to the enemy.

The months passed, the Allies won the war in Europe, and VE-day was joyfully celebrated on May 8, 1945. It was not long before word came through that our hospital unit would be broken up with the good news that we were going home for thirty days' leave. Following this, we were to reassemble at Fort Dix, New Jersey, and ship out to Camp Crowder, Missouri, for a month to form new hospitals and go to the Pacific Theater for the invasion of Japan.

Our remaining patients were transferred elsewhere, and our hospital was closed. The unit was divided into two groups, and the first one shipped out one week before my section. With joy and light hearts, we boarded the luxury liner, *Queen Elizabeth*, which was a troopship during the war. What had been a dream was coming true. I was going home!

After a pleasant five-day voyage, with no need to zigzag to avoid German submarines as on our trip to England, our ship entered New York Harbor. It was elating to set foot on American soil once again. Upon release, we said, "Goodbye, have a good time, see you in a month," to our buddies and headed home at the end of June 1945.

Chapter 13

The return home of a soldier in good physical and mental health after a tour of duty overseas, even if not exposed to combat, is a momentous occasion for a family. Knowing my leave was only for a month did not dampen our celebration.

I had previously informed my parents and sister about Blossom in a casual way. After getting settled, I talked about going to Lebanon to visit her. In our discussion, I learned that Schroon Lake was going to have a big Fourth of July celebration because of the European victory. Local soldiers who were home were to be the guests of honor.

My parents were quite excited by the fact that their son, who was now almost thirty-two years old, sounded serious about a girl. They suggested that the Fourth of July would be a wonderful time for her to visit us so we could meet, even though this was the busiest time of the year in our store.

On one of my calls to Blossom, I explained that under normal circumstances, I would visit her first. However, because of the Fourth of July celebration, I asked her if it would be possible for her to come to Schroon Lake first so we could get together and have her meet my family. She replied, "I'll have to ask my mother, I'll let you know."

The next time we spoke, the answer was yes. By this time, she had graduated from college and was working in the laboratory at Indiantown Gap, a nearby military installation. There must have been plenty of boyfriends in uniform because when her mother asked, "Which one is he?" The answer was, "The one who liked your sponge cake." Her mother happily gave the consent.

The visit was a huge success. Blossom, my parents, my sister and her husband, other family and friends all liked one another immediately. I knew I was in love from the first moment we got together, and she was strongly attracted to me. She was very comfortable with all of us, and we had a great time.

It dawned on me that Blossom was very much like my mother and sister, whom I idealized. Everyone approved of her and encouraged me in every way to make the most of our relationship. In normal times, I would have proposed, and we would have become engaged. Instead, although as lovesick as anyone could be, I agonized and hesitated, not so much for myself but for her future.

Would it be fair for a few weeks of wedded bliss to leave behind a lonely young wife who might end up a widow or married to a hopeless cripple or the mother of a child who might never know the father? Living alone at home with her parents, it would be like her life was ended before it really began. Also, selfishly on my part, I knew from observation in England that being overseas as a single man was far less stressful than as a husband. We did a lot of serious talking, but I did not propose.

We all had a wonderful time, and Blossom left for home. We were a perfect match, the opportunity of a lifetime—that was not to be at this time because of the war. It was a terribly frustrating, agonizing time for me.

Blossom and I kept in touch. Since my orders were for me to report to Fort Dix, New Jersey, on Saturday, August 4, 1945, I arranged to visit her in Lebanon from Thursday, August 2 until Saturday to say goodbye.

My plans were to visit some relatives in the New York City area on the way there, and my cousin helped me purchase a very nice compact as a gift for Blossom, something not too personal.

Before taking the train from Pennsylvania Station, I called a friend from the 93rd General Hospital who had reported to Fort Dix with the contingent who had left England one week ahead of me. He gave me the surprising news that all their orders had been changed, and no one was going to Camp Crowder to form a new hospital unit or go overseas. Instead, they were being dispersed individually to separate installations all over the United States. I sensed that if it happened to the first contingent, it would happen to mine.

There was a three-hour train ride to Ephrata, Pennsylvania, the station closest to Lebanon, which was another hour away by car. On that train ride, as I mulled over the astounding news from my buddy, a complete transformation in my thinking took place. A miracle had occurred. When Blossom picked me up, I would tell her the story about the change of events and propose that we get married right away so she could be with me when reporting to Fort Dix in two days.

After being picked up at the railroad station, I eagerly explained the anticipated completely changed outlook and proposed. The answer was yes, and by the time we arrived at her home in Lebanon, our minds were set on getting married the following day, if at all possible.

The next step was to break the news to her parents who were waiting to greet me, a soldier whom they had met just once before. They knew about Blossom's affection for me, but this was just going to be a two-day visit before my departure to prepare to go to the Pacific area for the invasion of Japan. It was the surprise of their lives when we walked in and announced our intention to get married the next day. They gave us their approval, and over lunch, we seriously discussed plans to arrange the seemingly impossible, our wedding tomorrow.

Blossom and her parents quickly impressed me with their organizing ability. Her father arranged to speak to a judge he knew to get the three-day waiting period waived and got this done. Now we were able to get a marriage license. Because of my military status, Blossom was able to get our blood tests done at Indiantown Gap, the nearby military installation where she worked. The results would be reported without delay.

She was also able to arrange for the Jewish chaplain on the post to perform the wedding the next day, Friday, rather late in the afternoon, by which time we hoped all the legal requirements would be completed.

Her mother then called family and friends, gave them the surprising news and invited them to attend the wedding. She also arranged details like flowers. Much to our surprise, in one day, she arranged a beautiful wedding dinner after the ceremony in our honor for family and friends at the famous Hershey Hotel in nearby Hershey, Pennsylvania.

All I knew about getting married was a wedding ring would be required. Blossom's cousin took me to a reliable jewelry store where a simple gold ring was purchased for her, but my dislike for wearing a ring ruled out a double-ring ceremony.

Thursday evening, in a call to my parents, they were told the exciting news. They were surprised, thrilled, and gave us their blessing. Mrs. Levitz spoke to them and urged them to come to the wedding, but it was not possible. My family's absence was the only negative element in the entire scenario, which came together in a lovely wedding ceremony in the military chapel on August 3, 1945. Still, there was some strangeness about the event where I would be meeting two of Blossom's brothers and their wives, family members, and friends for the first time.

Everything happened so fast that we were not able to find an available hotel room to spend our wedding night. Fortunately, my new in-laws owned a summer cottage a few miles outside of Lebanon where they lived in the summer. They moved back into town and gave us the cottage where we went after the dinner at the Hershey Hotel.

The next morning, Saturday, we had breakfast with Mother and Dad. They had just received a telegram from the military forwarded from Schroon Lake which told me my orders had been changed but reporting in at Fort Dix that day was still required. It was a wonderful wedding present. All of us were elated.

Soon after breakfast, my wife and I departed for Fort Dix, New Jersey, and an unknown future.

Chapter 14

Blossom and I were together when I reported in at Fort Dix on Saturday for a brief processing. No information was given me except to return on Monday morning for my assignment. It was to the headquarters of the Sixth Service Command in Omaha, Nebraska.

We discussed trying to get a leave for the purpose of getting our lives in order after the unexpected turn of events of the past few days.

A call was made to my new commanding officer asking for a delay en route (a leave) before reporting to him in Omaha. When I explained the situation, he granted me ten days.

We returned to Lebanon where Blossom gathered up clothes and personal belongings. Her parents arranged a wedding reception for us in their home to introduce me to their many family members and friends. Blossom's surprise wedding was the talk of the town, and everyone at the reception showered me with the highest compliments about her.

Then we headed for Schroon Lake and a joyous reception by the Friedmans who arranged for us to honeymoon in a lovely motel in town. Several relatives from the New York area were vacationing in town, and my parents arranged for a delightful family wedding dinner in a local restaurant. Time went much too quickly, and soon we were on the train to Omaha because we had no car.

My fairly new Ford car had been left at home when I went overseas. Foolishly, I told my parents to sell it when someone offered them a good price. At the time of our wedding, there were no cars to be had.

In Omaha, they had no assignment for me, so we continued to enjoy our honeymoon. During this time, the atomic bombs were dropped on Japan, and soon after, Japan surrendered. The war was over. Now it was understandable why my orders to go to Japan had been cancelled. From my standpoint, President Truman acted wisely and properly dropping the atomic bombs, since this act probably saved a million American lives, possibly mine.

My assignment was to the army post at Fort Leavenworth, Kansas. Because of the military, living quarters in town were at a premium. We succeeded in renting a room without kitchen privileges. A few weeks later, we rented a small apartment and furnished it with used furniture.

We obtained a car by a stroke of luck. Blossom's brother, Sidney, an army officer, had married a girl from Little Rock, Arkansas, in a hurry-up marriage there just before his transfer to California. Only his mother attended the wedding and had met the bride. They had a car on the West Coast from where Sid shipped out to the Pacific Theater in the army of occupation. His wife, Roberta, didn't need the car. Arrangements were made through family for it to be given to us. Roberta drove the car from the West Coast to Kansas City, where the three of us met for the first time.

Roberta was blond, with delicate, lovely facial features and a trim, slender body. Besides being so physically attractive, she was bright and a very warm personality. We immediately felt very comfortable with each other. After a short visit over lunch, we transferred the car and put her on a train to Little Rock, Arkansas. It was one of those unusual wartime experiences. For many years after the war, our families enjoyed numerous good times together.

A few days after we were comfortably at home in our apartment, I received orders to report immediately to the O'Reilly General Hospital in Springfield, Missouri, as head of the ear, nose, and throat department. We were separated for the first time because Blossom had to stay behind to find someone to take over our lease and buy our furniture. The demand for apartments was much greater than the supply, and she efficiently completed the process in a few days. She moved our belongings in our car and joined me.

There we found another apartment and settled in. This was my last assignment, and my discharge was delayed for a few months because no replacement could be found to take over my duties.

In the fall, my brother Moe was discharged from the army. He, my parents, my sister and her husband drove to Lebanon to meet Blossom's family for the first time. From there they drove to Springfield to visit us. We were delighted, and all had a wonderful time. Blossom and I were most happy to hear how very well our two families had hit it off on their visit.

I was now eligible to take the examination of the American Board of Otolaryngology and, if passed, to become a diplomate. This was very prestigious, since it meant that I had met all the training requirements to be recognized as a competent ear, nose, and throat specialist.

My instincts told me that my chances of passing this difficult examination would be better if it was taken while still in uniform. My application was submitted and accepted for the examination that was being given in Chicago in May 1946. Fortunately and happily, my discharge from the service occurred shortly before this time, so Chicago was a stop on our way to the East Coast, but wearing my uniform was still proper. It was a tough examination, and being in uniform didn't hurt. I did pass.

In retrospect, my army experience was a positive defining time in my life. First and foremost, meeting Blossom and marrying her was the best thing that ever happened to me. Professionally, most of my time had been spent working in my chosen field. During this time, my life changed from that of a student to a much more mature, traveled, and experienced worldly person. The horrors and carnage of war had been observed. My health was good. My professional and personal ethics and approach to relationships had been tested and served me well.

Blossom and I were very happy as we headed east to our families, with whom we would discuss and decide on our future plans.

Chapter 15

We now had to decide where to establish our home and my practice. I had always loved the upstate New York area where I spent my youth and obtained much of my education. Glens Falls and Albany were my first choices. Blossom also liked these locations. It seemed to me that Glens Falls was saturated with doctors in my field, and Albany appeared a better choice.

An affordable building was found in Albany suitable for a home and office in an excellent location. After purchasing it, repairs and alterations were made in the building. Equipment was acquired for my practice, which started in the fall of 1946.

I had friends in the medical community and the area. My first problem was obtaining hospital-staff appointments, which I found frustrating and was never resolved to my satisfaction, although my practice was growing.

Blossom became involved in the community, made many friends on her own, and we had an enjoyable social life. Our daughter Barbara was born on May 2, 1948.

It became obvious that the hospital situation was not going to improve in the near future to benefit me. This displeased me. Among the summer residents in Schroon Lake was a very successful older ear, nose, and throat specialist from Brooklyn. In a conversation with him, I told him about my unhappy situation. He told me he needed an assistant in his practice and offered me the position. After considerable further discussion with Blossom, our families, and Dr. Samuel Greenfield, with whom I would be associated, we came to an agreement. It was disappointing to feel the need to move, but it was accomplished quickly during the summer of 1948.

Dr. Greenfield's office was in the Eastern Parkway section of Brooklyn. We moved into a bright, comfortable upstairs apartment in a new two-family home occupied by the owner downstairs. Hospital privileges were quickly obtained at the Brooklyn Eye and Ear Hospital through Dr. Greenfield and at the Beth El Hospital because of my internship there.

Dr. Joseph Gilbert was the chief of service in Otolaryngology at the Kings County and Kingston Avenue city hospitals in Brooklyn. He also was on the staff at the Beth El Hospital and knew me as an intern there. He offered me a position as an attending surgeon in his department at the Kingston Avenue Hospital, which was devoted entirely to infectious diseases. Even though it was a public hospital, it was the only hospital in Brooklyn that accepted patients with all kinds of infectious diseases. Patients who otherwise would not go to a public hospital had to go to Kingston Avenue. I knew the volume and nature of the work there would be a challenging learning experience for a young surgeon like me.

I accepted this part-time volunteer appointment. An infantile paralysis (poliomyelitis) epidemic resulted in many patients with bulbar poliomyelitis, who required tracheotomy (an operation where a tube is inserted into the windpipe in the lower part of the neck). These patients could not breathe, and we had to provide an artificial airway before placing them in a respirator (iron lung).

I greatly enjoyed my volunteer service at the Kingston Avenue Hospital because the volume of patients requiring the specialized surgery done there could not be found in other hospitals.

In Brooklyn at that time, a great deal of surgery, like tonsillectomies and nasal operations, was performed in doctors' offices. We had very well-equipped facilities in our office, and much surgery was done there.

We had family in the area, found friends, and were enjoying our life as a family. I was busy and happier than in Albany. Our daughter Beverly was born on April 28, 1950. Among my cousins in Brooklyn was Fanny James, somewhat older than us and a personable, attractive, bright woman. She and Blossom became very close friends, and because Fanny's husband wasn't home much, she spent a good deal of time with us and adored our children.

The following "truth is stranger than fiction" story occurred because of her. I had purchased a new car in Manhattan and had an afternoon free to go pick it up and leave my trade-in. Blossom was busy with the children. Fanny was good company, so I asked her to join me for the ride, and she liked the idea. When we arrived at the dealership, we were disappointed to hear that it would be a few hours before the car would be ready. It didn't make sense to drive home and come back. Blossom was called and told why we would be late returning. Since we had enough time for the show at Radio City, we decided to go there.

During our summers on the beach in Schroon Lake as newlyweds, Blossom and I had become friendly with an actress, who had starred in a Broadway play. As Fanny and I entered the theater lobby, we met her coming out. We recognized and greeted each other, and I introduced my attractive, well-dressed companion as my "cousin." She thought she got the message, didn't ask any questions that might be embarrassing, and moved on quickly. We had a good laugh when the implications were explained to Fanny at the time and to Blossom when we arrived home. Years later, our guide in Italy would point out every good-looking girl as his "cousin," which kept reminding me of this incident.

After a few years, Dr. Greenfield was anxious to retire and sell me his home-office building and practice. By this time, Blossom and I were questioning whether we wanted to live and bring up our children in Brooklyn. When we tried to go to Jones Beach, we usually were hung up in horrendous traffic and might not even get there in time to enjoy it. This was just a single example where our small-town memories told us things could be better. On the other hand, we enjoyed the cultural advantages, like Broadway shows, the New York City Ballet, and the museums.

The area where we had our office was changing and appeared to be in decline. From the long-range view, the practice did not appeal to me. We decided that if we moved again, it would be to a small community.

I began to look at advertisements in the medical journals, and to my surprise, in the summer of 1951, there was an advertisement offering an ear, nose, and throat practice for sale in Glens Falls. A call was placed immediately to answer the advertisement, and it was determined that the doctor was seriously ill and would never practice again. This appeared like the opportunity of a lifetime, and without delay, I arranged a visit to look into the situation.

Chapter 16

Of course, Glens Falls was familiar territory. The ill doctor was in a hospital about three hours away, but I had made an appointment with his secretary-aide to look at the office and speak to her. On arriving there and making introductions, we recognized each other as high-school classmates.

The office was in an office building and was quite well equipped. I found out that there was no longer an active practice, and taking it over meant almost starting anew. Surprisingly, he was the only physician in town practicing allergy, a recent trend among ear, nose, and throat specialists.

Inquiries about a hospital-staff appointment and the practice opportunity had been favorable.

The owner of the practice was able to talk and negotiate, and I went to visit him. We agreed on a price for the equipment. I would assume his lease. The deal was set, and his lawyers would handle the completion of the sale.

I also made courtesy calls on the other two specialists in my field and introduced myself.

It would be at least six weeks before actually being able to start in Glens Falls. I was working without a contract and gave my notice to Dr. Greenfield. I continued with him in order to fulfill my obligations.

To be able to practice allergy would be an important asset, and I soon enrolled in the best intensive course in allergy available, which happened to be in New York City. The course was excellent and gave me the needed knowledge, preparation, and confidence to include the field of allergy in my new practice.

We found an apartment in Glens Falls in which to live. The move was in October 1951. I was home.

I knew on coming there that the surgical department of the Glens Falls Hospital had a rule that a new member could not perform any surgery for six months. It was very unfair, and Dr. Edmunds, the head of our department, told me not to worry, that I could admit my patients under his name and do the operations myself. This was a fine gesture on his part, and we became good friends.

However, this was breaking the rules. One prejudiced person could give me a hard time when my name came up for an attending appointment after six months. As difficult as it was for me, I decided to only admit emergency patients on Dr. Edmund's service to be operated upon by me.

We settled into the community and time passed slowly, doing only office practice. When March rolled around, my wait for surgical privileges should have been over. I received a call from Dr. Maslon, the chief of staff, telling me that the committee could not meet that month because of a lack of a quorum to make the appointment, that it was merely a formality now and would happen next month.

It may have been a formality to others, but to me it was a big disappointment, especially since I had patients waiting for elective operations like tonsillectomies and adenoidectomies. Blossom and I decided that the best thing to do was take a vacation in Miami Beach, Florida, for a couple of weeks. Her parents were there, and they found us a desirable place to stay with our two children. Blossom had been to Florida once before, but it was my first time in this winter paradise.

The vacation on the beach was very relaxing and, spending time with family, enjoyable. It proved to be a smart move. Soon after returning home, I was awarded a hospital-staff appointment, and my career took off.

Our third and last child, our son Victor, was born on December 28, 1952.

We began to think about building a home and, in 1954, bought a lot that was desirable at a bargain price. No one wanted the property because it was next to a gasoline station but separated by dense woods. In our estimation, the gas station would not detract from our home, and time proved we were correct. When the owner of the business died a few years later, the building was torn down, and we bought the adjacent wooded area.

We started to look at architectural magazines for a house plan for our property. Eventually, we found a plan that looked ideal for our lot. Blossom was gifted with artistic and architectural vision. When she looked at a certain plan, she knew immediately that this was the perfect plan for us. She also said, "It has a door leading from the kitchen which would make a perfect connection for an entrance from the house to the office if you would ever want to add one on to our home." At that time, a home-office was the last thing in my mind.

She was enthusiastic about the split-level plan, but lacking her vision, I wanted to see the house before making a decision. I called the magazine, and they gave me a location on Long Island where a group of the houses had been built. We visited the area and were impressed with their outside appearance. While looking around, we were invited inside by a family when we explained why we were there. They were very happy with the plan and even told us where it could be improved. It was very kind and helpful of them, and we sent them a gift and letter of appreciation.

We were sold on the house and sent for the blueprints which cost $35.00, our total architectural expense. We had already told the best home-building contractor in the area, Lloyd Kingsley, that we wanted him to build our home. We showed him the blueprints, and he agreed it was an excellent plan for our lot and purposes. There were some modifications that Blossom wanted to make, and together they worked them out.

Mr. Kingsley lived up to his reputation. It was a pleasure to work with him. There were never any serious problems, since he kept his word on everything. For us, building was an enjoyable experience. In 1955, we moved into our new home, which was all we hoped it would be.

Chapter 17

Moving into our new home was a milestone in the progress of the Orel Friedman family toward living the American Dream. Blossom and I were in a happy marriage with three healthy children. My practice was successful and growing.

We joined the Reform temple in Glens Falls, Temple Beth El, and met many young couples with young families like ours, which resulted in becoming involved in an active and enjoyable social and religious life. Blossom's leadership ability and talent had quickly been recognized, and from 1955 to 1957, she served as president of the Glens Falls Chapter of Hadassah, the Women's Zionist Organization of America. She loved the causes it supported and devoted much of her life working as a volunteer eventually rising to the highest level, the National Board.

We also were active in temple leadership and activities relating to Israel. Over the course of many years, I was on the committee and served as chairman of the United Jewish Appeal and Israel Bond fund drives.

All four of our parents were living; they were very compatible. And for a few years, our parents, our family and other relatives spent the Jewish High Holidays together in a hotel in Saratoga Springs. Blossom had four brothers and two sisters, while I had a sister and a brother. We had many aunts, uncles, and cousins on both sides of the family, with whom we and our children spent many happy times.

Schroon Lake, about forty miles from Glens Falls, was a frequent destination for swimming, boating, and water skiing, the latter for the children. After Moe and his wife, Janet, bought a camp on the east side of Schroon Lake, we had many wonderful parties there. My parents loved all these lakeside parties with children, grandchildren, and many friends around them.

During the summers, Blossom would drive the children to Lebanon, Pennsylvania, her hometown, to visit her parents and family without me because I had to work. Occasionally, I accompanied them.

To be truthful, I looked forward to the temporary aloneness. It was having rare quality time on my own to do some serious thinking, catch up on neglected matters, and relax. I didn't want to appear ungrateful to my many well-meaning friends who showered me with dinner invitations so I wouldn't be lonely, but in time, I succeeded in avoiding being entertained. Although I am a social animal, enjoying aloneness at times is very important to me. Later in life, this was a defining factor in my successful adjustment as a widower.

When possible, however, we took many family trips together. The highlight was flying to California in the early 1960s to visit Disneyland, go sightseeing, and look up family.

Both Blossom and I loved to travel, and in the 1960s, we began to take trips to interesting places in the United States and abroad, usually where there was a medical meeting. In 1965, we went on a three-week trip to Japan and Hong Kong to attend an international meeting in my specialty. Japan was one of most enjoyable places we ever visited. We also began taking trips to Israel. We were fortunate in finding reliable women to look after our children while we were away. When the children were older, our very good friends, the Forrests, took them into their home in our absence. We reciprocated by doing the same for the Forrest children when their parents took a vacation. It was an excellent arrangement.

To add to the international flavor of our lives, a very bright, attractive, and personable Italian exchange student, Daniella, on an American Field Service Program, lived in our home for a school year, 1963 to 1964. It was a wonderful experience for all of us. A few years later, after Daniella was married, Blossom and I visited her and her husband in Italy and also met her parents and brother. Early in 2001, my son Victor was in Italy and visited her.

It was on this trip to Italy that we discovered, on the day of our departure, that our passports had expired. How we obtained passports and made our flight was a thrilling story. My intent was to write the story and get it published. When I started writing, it was clear to me the tools were lacking. Our community college gave an excellent course in creative writing. Enrolling in this program was a revelation and very beneficial. The story was eventually written but never was accepted for publication.

In different years, our children, Barbara and Victor, spent their junior year in high school as exchange students attending a high school in Haifa, Israel, sponsored by the Reform Religious Movement. They lived with Israeli families and nurtured their growing interest in the Jewish state.

Our daughter Beverly was quite rebellious, and against her wishes, we decided that living away from home in a boarding school would best promote her development and education. Fortunately, we chose the Stockbridge School in Massachusetts, which proved to be the kind of school she needed. In time, she made the necessary adjustments and graduated with her Stockbridge class.

Barbara graduated from the Glens Falls High School in 1966 and entered Brandeis University that fall, majoring in Near East and Judaic Studies and a premedical course. There she met Terry Plasse from Great Neck, New York, who graduated in the class of 1969, one year ahead of Barbara. They became engaged that summer, and in the fall, he entered the Washington University School of Medicine in St. Louis. Barbara completed her requirements for graduation at midterm, and on February 1, 1970, they were married in a large, beautiful wedding attended by family members and friends from all over the country.

Barbara and Terry lived in St. Louis until his graduation in 1973. She never went to medical school but earned a master's degree in social work and became a registered nurse (RN) there. They then moved to New York City where Terry was a resident in internal medicine (Beth Israel Hospital) and later a fellow in oncology (the study of tumors) at Mt. Sinai Hospital. They remained in New York and live there now.

Chapter 18

Our daughter Beverly graduated from the Stockbridge School in 1968 and, in the fall, enrolled in the four-year nursing program at Boston University, leading to the degree of Bachelor of Science in Nursing. She enjoyed the program, did very well, and, in her senior year, worked part time as a nurse. After graduation, she began working full time as a nurse at the university hospital. In the late fall, she went to Europe to visit some European students she had met and become friendly with in Boston.

From Europe, she continued on to Israel. In her earlier years, she had not been interested in Israel, in contrast to Barbara and Victor. While in college, she had joined a youth mission to the Jewish state and was now fulfilling her desire to return there.

In January 1973, Beverly enrolled in a one-year program sponsored by the World Union of Jewish Students (WUJIS) for college graduates from other countries for the purpose of encouraging them to immigrate to Israel. The first six months were spent studying the Hebrew language, Jewish culture and traditions, and becoming informed about the state of Israel. The second six months were to be spent in a work program utilizing the students' educational skills.

A classmate was a young man, Joel Seligson, from Finland, where there was a small, decreasing Jewish population. He wanted to live an active Jewish life and enrolled in the WUJIS program after graduating from Helsinki University with a degree in optical physics. For both of them, it must have been "love at first sight."

His parents visited Israel early in the year, met Beverly, and, apparently, were impressed. We went to Israel in April to visit her and met Joel, whom we liked very much. By this time, it was obvious that they were serious about each other. They were happy that both sets of parents had been there and approved of their choices.

Their goal for the work program was to spend it together utilizing their different skills. Unfortunately, this didn't work out, and they were unhappy to the extent that they were planning to leave the program and Israel. This meant they would separate from each other and return to their homes.

Joel's father was the manager of the table-tennis team from Finland competing in the Maccabi Games (so-called Jewish Olympics) in Israel that summer. When he saw them and heard their story, to keep them from breaking up, he invited Beverly and Joel to return to Finland with him on the team plane and spend time together in the Seligson home. Beverly and Joel accepted the offer.

Joel's parents, Lilli and Boris Seligson, were fluent in English, worldly, and understanding. They liked the match and encouraged it. Before long, Blossom received a call from Beverly telling us that they wanted to get married. It was a surprise, and Blossom was somewhat skeptical until Lilli came on the phone, introduced herself, told us how wonderful Beverly was, and confirmed what had been said.

She wanted to get married in Glens Falls, and the only weekend convenient for the Seligsons to come for the wedding was September 21 to 23, 1973. There was a conclave of children scheduled at our Temple Beth El that weekend, which ruled out using it. We decided to have the wedding at the beautiful Glens Falls Country Club, to which we belonged. All went well, and Beverly and Joel were married in a joyful, traditional manner. We were happy to meet Joel's parents who stayed at our home. The newlyweds returned to Helsinki, Finland, where Joel entered graduate school. Beverly learned Finnish rapidly and soon was working as a nurse anesthetist in a hospital.

There was a visiting professor at Helsinki University from the University of Rochester in Rochester, New York, in the Department of Optical Physics, Joel's field of study. He recognized Joel's ability and offered him full scholarships to attend the University of Rochester to obtain a Ph.D.

Joel eagerly accepted this wonderful opportunity, and in 1975, they moved to Rochester where Joel continued his education and Beverly started working as a nurse.

Chapter 19

Our son Victor was always a dreamer. One day, I found him daydreaming and asked, "Why are you sitting there doing nothing?"

His reply was, "Dad, I need time to think."

He was serious in giving me this answer, and time has proven that he was on the right track. A defining moment in his development occurred when he went to a summer camp at Warwick, New York, sponsored by the Union of American Hebrew Congregations, the Reform movement. There he met Jewish contemporaries who had excellent religious backgrounds. Realizing how inadequate his religious knowledge was, he decided to work and study hard until he was their equal. He did this and developed an intellectual and emotional love for Judaism which has persisted until this day.

High school was not very challenging, and the opportunity to spend the junior school year in Israel was most welcome. His one athletic accomplishment in high school was to make the swimming team, a sport in which he continues to excel.

He entered Brandeis University in their Middle East and Judaic Studies Program, which he found challenging, and became proficient in Hebrew and Arabic. He did well and was elected to the Phi Beta Kappa Society. There he met Thomas L. Friedman, now a renowned author and columnist for *The New York Times*, with whom he has had a lifelong friendship.

During his college years, he explored all the different Jewish religious sects and opted to become very traditional in his observance of Judaism.

In the intervening years, until his marriage in 1979, Victor spent one year studying in a yeshiva, an Orthodox religious school, and decided that their lifestyle was not for him. He took a job teaching English in an Arab high school in Masada in the Golan Heights, the northern area of the country won from Syria in the 1967 war. It was a very positive experience. Although the only Jewish teacher in the school, his students and Arab faculty found him exceptionally competent and likeable. He was fond of the Arab culture and was very happy there, establishing friendships that existed for many years. However, he was not allowed to live in this all-Arab community and had to commute to work daily by taxi.

Blossom and I visited him in the summer of 1977 and were treated royally by his students and their families. We stayed on a kibbutz, Neve Ativ, which, in the winter, served as a hotel for skiers on Mt. Hermon, a ski area on the Golan Heights. Except for breakfast, we ate all our meals as guests in Arab homes for four days. Most everyone in the four villages served by the school, three Druze villages and one Alawite Muslim village, wanted to entertain us, so they drew lots in each village to pick those homes where we were guests. Usually, the women served their men and us but didn't eat with us. It was a happy, memorable experience. Although much of the food was strange to us, there were no ill effects. The school also put on a party in honor of Victor and his parents.

In the fall of 1977, Victor met Nurit Levi, a sabra (a native-born Israeli) and graduate of Hebrew University working as a counselor for American college graduates doing volunteer work in Israel. It was the beginning of a romance between an Israeli of Yemenite descent and an American whose grandparents came from Eastern Europe.

They were married on July 9, 1979, in a traditional ceremony at a restaurant catering to such functions on the Tower of David in Jerusalem. Nurit's parents and their large extended family lived close to one another in a small city called Zichron Yaakov, which means "Remember Jacob" (Rothschild), a philanthropist who supported the early settlers. It is a lovely, picturesque city located on a bluff overlooking the Mediterranean Sea. Nurit's parents also became our good friends.

The newlyweds came to the United States in November 1979. Victor went to Columbia University Teachers College in New York

City. His studies were in applied human development and guidance. He was awarded a master of arts (MA) degree from Columbia University in 1981. From there he went to Harvard University, where, in 1986, he received a doctor of education degree (EdD) in counseling, consulting, and community psychology.

Nurit's degree was in mathematics and statistics, and she found employment at Mt. Sinai Hospital in New York in the field of medical statistics. She proved to be very innovative and competent. When they moved to the Boston area, Nurit went to work for a company with a handful of employees in the new field of medical cost-effective studies. The company prospered and, five years later, had 150 employees, and Nurit was in charge of about 40 of them.

At this point in our lives, Blossom and I were the happy parents of three married children who were starting their own families and giving us the gift of grandchildren. They all lived about a four-hour drive from Glens Falls and visited us as often as possible. Our home was centrally located, large, and the perfect meeting place for the many happy times we enjoyed as a family. Many gatherings were hosted by my brother's family, who loved to entertain at their cottage on the east side of Schroon Lake. Our close friends, the Busmans, also had great parties for us at their ideally located, comfortable home and grounds on the shore of famous Lake George.

Over the years, our happiness was marred by the deaths of our parents, who had shared many of the good times with us. Otherwise, it was the best of times.

Chapter 20

After a few years in Glens Falls, my practice had grown to the extent that the office I had taken over in 1951 was becoming inadequate for my needs. It might have been possible to expand the existing office, but the building was being neglected by the landlord. This disturbed me so much that I began to dislike entering the building and felt that the conditions were disrespectful to my patients.

After several futile attempts to arrange to build an office building with other doctors, Blossom encouraged me to build an office as an addition to our home that would be attached but otherwise completely separate. The location was perfect, since our corner lot faced the main street where there were existing professional offices. The entrance to our home faced the side street, and our privacy would not be compromised. She had visualized all this ten years earlier when we chose the plan for our home. In her wisdom, she convinced me this was the best solution to a new office.

For several years, I had been interested in medical-office planning and, from personal experience, knew precisely what my needs and those of my patients would be. At one of our national professional meetings, a course was given on office planning for our specialty by a local doctor, who even showed us his office. My impression was that it could be improved upon for my needs.

Blossom and I then drew up our plan for the office in which we included the first sound-proof room for hearing testing in our area and heavy wiring for an X-ray machine and any future needs. We then gave our plan to an architect for refinement and to be made into blueprints. Lloyd Kingsley, our builder, again did a magnificent job, and in 1965, I moved into my new office. It was extremely efficient to work in and comfortably supportive and considerate of the needs of my patients. It was known as a showplace. There was a door that led from our kitchen to the office, the only connection, just as Blossom had visualized it ten years earlier. Otherwise, they were two separate buildings. I loved my new office.

By this time, you know Blossom was someone outstanding. Her siblings were of the same caliber, and in the 1970s, her family name, Levitz, became nationally famous when two of her brothers, Ralph and Leon, established the Levitz Furniture Corporation, a nationwide chain of stores which revolutionized the retail furniture industry. They introduced the warehouse concept, whereby, if you wished, you could choose the furniture you wanted in their spacious showroom, immediately pick it up from the attached large warehouse, truck it home yourself in your own vehicle, and save a lot of money. The company prospered, went public, and for a while, their stock soared.

Of the immediate family, we were the only ones not involved in the furniture business. For quite a few years, the family enjoyed exciting, heady times. Some members of the family became very wealthy. We held some stock, but unfortunately, eventually, the bubble burst, and I continued making my living the old-fashioned way by working at my profession.

It was our good fortune to have children who married young and started their own families early before they were established in careers. For this, I have always felt indebted to them because my age was fifty-nine and Blossom's fifty-two when Amitai Plasse was born in 1973. Then came Ori Plasse in 1975; Michal Seligson, 1977; Eitan Plasse, 1978; Miriam Seligson, 1978; Nomi Friedman, 1981; Haviva Seligson, 1981; Ayala Seligson, 1982; Micah Friedman, 1984; and Gilead Friedman, 1987. They were all born in the United States, and our eleventh grandchild, Tamar Friedman, was born in Israel in 1989. We greatly enjoyed our grandparenting, and my retirement in 1980 was a blessing in this regard, since it gave us much more time and freedom to travel and spend time with family.

Another way in which our children brought happiness into our lives was through their marriages, all of which have stood the test of time so far.

Sherley and Herman Plasse, Terry's parents, became our very good friends, and their home in Great Neck, New York, was always open to us (and it seems like everyone we knew or were related to). They loved to entertain, and their friends became our friends. One of Sherley's best friends with whom we became close is Ruth Popkin, a former national president of Hadassah and at one time the most important woman in Jewish life in the world. We and the Plasses visited each other often, and they came to Israel several times to be with us on holidays and celebrations after Beverly and Victor and their families moved to Israel.

Joel's parents, Lilli and Boris Seligson, also became our very good friends. We visited them once in Finland, and they visited us a few times. We spent a delightful vacation on Cape Cod together. On another occasion, Janet and Moe threw a big birthday party for Lilli at their rustic lakeshore cottage on Schroon Lake. Her North American relatives from all over were invited, and it seems the partying went on for about four days. We also were together several times in Israel.

The Seligsons' close friends, Rosemarie and Leo Millner, who live in Tel Aviv, Israel, became our good friends. When our son Victor was teaching in the Golan Heights, he became seriously ill with hepatitis. The only people he knew well enough in Israel to ask for help were the Millners. Rosemarie was an operating-room nurse in Tel Aviv and arranged for his hospitalization and care. She and Leo saw that he received the best of care, kept us informed, and told us he was recovering favorably. After his discharge from the hospital, they took him into their home until he was completely well. They suggested we wait until he recovered to visit so we could really enjoy a little vacation together. We followed their advice and did just that.

Nurit's parents, Saadia and Margalit Levi, in Israel, were always very warm and cordial, and we also became good friends with them and their large extended family. Nurit's mother is a fabulous cook and baker, and whenever we came to visit Victor's family, they developed what was called a "magic refrigerator." Suddenly, it was stocked with all kinds of delicious cooked foods and pastries. Her mother made sure we would not go hungry.

We were fortunate that all these interpersonal relationships went so well over the years.

During the years before my retirement, our immediate family experienced numerous health problems. My hearing loss increased to the extent that in the 1950s, I began wearing a hearing aid. Having a hearing loss enabled me to empathize with my patients and their hearing problems. Many patients with hearing losses came to me for this reason. Mine is a hereditary type of nerve deafness and has affected some of my children and grandchildren.

Over the years, I suffered from low back pain which required hospitalization on two occasions and incapacitated me at home several times. Whatever the cause, it always responded to conservative therapy. In 1975, a superficial malignant melanoma was removed from my back and has not recurred. In 1978, I had a transurethral prostatic resection for benign prostatic hypertrophy. In 1979, severe hyperthyroidism incapacitated me to the extent that I performed no surgery for about six months.

In 1965, Blossom had a subtotal gastric resection for a chronic duodenal ulcer with an excellent result. In 1973, a kidney stone became lodged in her ureter, causing excruciating pain, which required a delicate operation called an ureterotomy for removal. She also had a hysterectomy, the removal of the uterus. Blossom always recovered quickly from surgery and remained very active.

It took many months for me to recover completely after treatment of my hyperthyroidism with radioactive isotopes. By the beginning of 1980, I was feeling well, and my practice was very active when, in April, the double vision occurred, which would change my life forever.

PART II

Chapter 21

Part 1 began with the events leading up to my unexpected and unplanned-for retirement and was followed by my life story from its beginning until my vision failed me.

This is a quote from chapter 4, "the feeling was that my life was over, but fortunately, it was only temporarily on hold. This is the story of a new beginning. Since every new beginning must start with an ending, it is necessary to familiarize you with the first sixty-six years of the life that had come to a halt." This was done in part 1.

Part 2 deals with the next twenty-five years of my life after retiring from medicine. The new beginning is explained very well by the following statement, "Wherever a man finds himself, there is a way by which he came and a way by which he can leave."(1)

The way I left this low point in my life to find happiness, growth as a personality, and fulfillment has been an intellectual and spiritual journey which evolved gradually over the years.

The previous month, April 1980, from the onset of my disability to my retirement, had been hectic with my staff and myself devoting ourselves to the tasks that had to be taken care of immediately. Anything nonessential was left for a later time.

Therefore, my secretary, who continued to work part time, and I were busy "mopping up" the details required in terminating a practice. Patients were still claiming their records and seeking referrals to other doctors. Insurance forms needed completion; bills had to be sent out and collected. Individuals and organizations had to be notified that my practice was closed.

---

[1]   *Hadassah Magazine*, December 2000, p. 114. This article was a review of the book *Sacrifice* by Todd Gitlin, 1999 by Todd Gitlin. Reprinted by arrangement with Henry Holt and Company, LLC.

Since I was hoping that another otolaryngologist would be interested in taking over my office and practice in the near future while there was still an active patient base to be transferred, much of my effort was devoted to this purpose. Advertisements were placed in medical journals, and personal contact was made with acquaintances and the directors of residency training services.

As a result of my retirement, there was also an excellent opportunity for an allergist in Glens Falls. A colleague in general practice also had a subspecialty practice in allergy, but there was a need for a full-time doctor in this field. Advertisements were also placed in allergy journals in an attempt to attract someone.

It did not take long for me to discover that the home-office arrangement which had made me and my family very happy would be a detriment rather than an attraction. It was a time of affluence, and the trend for most doctors and other professionals was to have a home in a desirable residential neighborhood and an office elsewhere suitable for that purpose. Also, the trend was changing rapidly from solo practices to group practices, and a home-office did not lend itself to the group concept. My setup had become an anachronism. This loss of innocence soon changed my approach to any inquiries and prospects.

Since we loved our large spacious home, which was central to our growing family for get-togethers, Blossom and I realized it would be financially feasible to stay there if an income was realized from the office. In talking to prospects, while emphasizing that the real estate and practice were for sale as a package, I could be flexible to the extent of selling my equipment and renting the office or even renting the office with the equipment. Realistically, for someone starting in practice, the purchase of expensive real estate and the office equipment could be scary.

The advantage was with a minimal outlay of funds, the entire office package could be made available immediately with a patient base from which to start. To sweeten the deal, I was not interested in selling "good will" or the practice, only the furniture and equipment. It was an offer that seemed to me an otolaryngologist could not refuse, but to my disappointment, it was.

In dealing with allergists who responded to my advertisements, I offered them the office, furnishings, and any equipment they desired. I also felt that if too much time did not pass, my allergy patients would return to the occupant of my office.

It was discouraging as months passed without any progress despite the fact that every lead was diligently followed-up corresponding and telephoning. At a later time, when discarding old correspondence, it was amazing to see how many letters were in my files and how many prospects had been contacted. My secretary was not needed for very long after my retirement, but fortunately, I am a good typist, and one of my hobbies has always been letter writing. Being occupied with this effort was probably good for me but frustrating.

There was an allergist, completing a fellowship in the Midwest, who responded to my advertisement and was very interested in coming to Glens Falls. We had a date for a visit. However, he was going to an allergy meeting in Las Vegas before coming here. The hotel he was staying at had a dangerous fire, and he barely escaped alive and lost everything he had in the hotel.

This was national news, and I read about the fire in the paper but did not relate the incident to him. A few days later, this young doctor called me and told me the horrible story. He was so badly traumatized at the time that he cancelled the visit. He promised to get back to me later, but he never did.

A Canadian allergist who was disillusioned with the medical system there showed great interest in my office. When questioned about licensing at his first visit, he assured me that he had investigated the matter and there would be no problem. It appeared that a deal was at hand, but at the last minute, he called to inform me that he was wrong about the licensing. There were definite roadblocks that had discouraged him from making the change.

Despite my herculean efforts eight months after closing my office, the end of 1980 rolled around with my office still empty, my real estate unsold, my practice having dwindled away. Although there were still inquiries, the situation appeared bleak. I kept up my advertising and effort, and ironically, I proved to be a great recruiter for the hospital and community. Before the next year would be over, both an otolaryngologist and an allergist whom I recruited started practices in Glens Falls. Neither, however, was interested in my real estate or office.

Chapter 22

In the previous chapter, the description of my lack of success disposing of my office and real estate was discouraging and depressing. Of even greater personal importance was my disengagement from the practice of medicine and my professional life, the center of my activity for so many years.

The expression "It is easy to quit smoking, I've done it a thousand times" comes to mind. Something can be easy if there are no roadblocks to returning to one's previous activity.

Even though for me there could be no turning back to my medical practice, disengagement on a conscious level was relatively easy. My office was closed with a sigh of relief because as a physically impaired physician, my comfort level was poor. Although all surgery had been discontinued and my office practice was limited to a minimum of procedures necessary to responsibly look after and close out my previous patient relationships, I was apprehensive.

Frankly, once my decision was made to retire, my desire was to get out as soon as possible without anything happening to tarnish the excellent reputation established during my years in the medical community. Until recently, I really enjoyed the practice of medicine, but now it had ceased to be "fun." There was definitely a feeling of relief.

My disability acted as a "wake up" call to bring to my attention that the inevitable end to my career had come much sooner than expected without any preparation for the change. At age sixty-six, a surgical career has a limited future. However, in otolaryngology and allergy, an office practice can be projected to continue well into the future. All these plans needed to be abandoned.

It was ended, and there was no straddling the fence looking back. It even amazed me how, on a conscious level, I seemed to disengage from my past.

On a subconscious level, however, it was different. For many years in my dreams, I was busy operating. Night after night was spent performing surgery. Some of the dreams were nightmares where I found myself in impossible situations only relieved by waking up. It took a long time to disengage from these thoughts submerged in my mind, but eventually it occurred.

What made the operating room (OR) so important that in my subconscious I could not let go? My concept of the OR is a very exclusive club where only a few people belong who are dedicated to the betterment of the lives of other men, women, and children by performing necessary skillful surgery. We are entrusted with the most valuable possession that people have: their lives and the lives of their families. Members of this club are the surgeons, nurses, members of the anesthesiology department, recovery-room personnel, the aides and maids. Working together closely day after day over the years under all kinds of crises and circumstances, we get to know one another extremely well. Teamwork is the essence of success, and adaptation to differing egos, temperaments, and personalities is necessary. Most importantly, what goes on in the OR should not be a source for gossip.

My approach to the nurses and other personnel in the OR was no different from the way my interpersonal relationships are conducted wherever I am. Everyone was treated with respect and consideration, and this was reciprocated. Under appropriate circumstances, I was known to tell jokes while operating, and my OR was a "happy" place to work. There were rumors that in the old days, some of the surgeons were not happy unless they left at least one nurse crying by the end of the day because of abuse. Times have changed.

There is something "stuffy" in my personality, and in contrast to many of the surgeons, my way of addressing the nurses was to use Miss or Mrs., rarely by their first names. It worked well for me, and there was mutual respect. Even when working with the most experienced personnel, when specialized instruments were needed for a procedure like a bronchoscopy for a foreign body in the lung, I always picked out the specialized instruments myself to be sure they were working properly and would be available when needed. If anything did not go smoothly, I wanted it to be my responsibility.

If, in a routine type of procedure, the use of a special instrument or piece of equipment might be needed, I would tell the nurse in advance to include it in the setup. Before starting the operation, I would ask if the special item was there. Even though the answer was yes, I would always say, "Let me see it." Seeing it made me feel comfortable knowing what was needed would be available. One can be thorough and responsible without being offensive or causing resentment.

Fortunately, in my field of practice, there was the satisfaction in a vast majority of patients of seeing positive results from the surgery in a relatively short time. Also, children undergoing tonsil and adenoid surgery and/or the placement of ventilating tubes in their ears were a big part of my practice. Working with children was especially pleasurable, and we related well to one another.

No wonder my life spent working in what was deemed a very special exclusive club kept recurring in my dreams for a long time after it was over.

As best I could, I made the rounds of my friends and associates to say "farewell" from the professional standpoint.

To my pleasant surprise a few weeks later, I received a telephone call from one of the OR nurses inviting my wife and me to a party in our honor in the nurses' lounge in the OR. It was a wonderful, sincere expression of their regard for me. Something I have appreciated, cherished, and remembered to this very day.

To top everything off, the nurses presented me with the gift of a collage they had made of two of my favorite instruments which had been changed in color to bronze to fit in with the brownish color scheme, dried flowers, and a poem written by the poet laureate of the OR, Kathy. It says:

Our O.R. suite,
just isn't the same.
We think of you often,
and mention your name.

And laugh aloud,
recalling the fun.
With tonsils and adenoids,
bad times there were none.

The afternoons', oh yes
so many did pass by.
Your little people knew,
there was no need to cry.

Your mannerism was kind,
your voice was so low.
The patients were ready,
Always ready to go.

We miss this man,
we consider a friend
But fond memories of you,
shall never, never end.

Our best to you,
And your lovely wife.
May you have peace and enjoyment,
the rest of your life.

Your O.R. Friends

This party came at a time when my mood was on the downside. Its effect was encouraging because it told me that I had been doing something right previously and there was no reason for my approach to life to change. This event definitely bolstered my morale, and the gift is greatly treasured and hangs in my den to be enjoyed daily.

Chapter 23

When it appeared that retirement was the only way out of my visual and practice dilemma, the realization that we faced a possible financial disaster was scary. Except for bills that were owed me by patients and insurance companies, the income from my practice would end abruptly. My professional expenses would diminish considerably but not entirely in the beginning.

How would we meet our obligations? Fortunately, we had lived within our means and were not in debt. Our home-office had no mortgage. For many years, I had carried a limited amount of disability insurance hoping it would never have to be used. My ophthalmologist assured me that he would certify I was completely disabled from a practice standpoint. This insurance proved to be a very helpful cushion at first.

I was eligible for Social Security and began collecting it. Blossom was eight years younger than I and not yet eligible for Social Security. Disbursements were taken from my Keough and IRA Plans. Blossom had small Keough and IRA Plans and would be eligible for disbursements by the end of the year. We also had a limited amount of income from investments.

We tried to cut down on our expenses, which proved to be rather difficult. When one of our two cars needed replacement, we decided to get along with one car since I was home much of the time. This led to some inconvenience, but we were respectful of each others needs, and it worked. In an emergency, a taxicab could be called. We both liked to walk. Downtown, especially the library, was twenty minutes from home. I enjoyed the walk both ways, and it was good exercise which I needed. Because of my double vision, I found it frustrating to try to hit a golf ball and had to stop playing. Walking a good deal was a blessing.

Resting my eyes was very beneficial, and my double vision gradually improved to a degree that with the incorporation of prisms in my corrective lenses (glasses), I could function fairly well.

Since there had been no preparation for my retirement, I was motivated to try to find out what retirement meant. The Crandall Library was a "gold mine" of books on the subject. In the course of time, most of the books in the collection about retirement were read. This stimulated my interest in gerontology, the field of study devoted to the aging. The library also contained a good collection on this subject which was read and proved informative. Many worthwhile hours were spent in the library.

At this particular time, the "gold bugs" were dominating the financial news. Their belief was that investments based on paper holdings like stocks, bonds, and bank accounts would be wiped out by a soon-to-arrive high inflationary spiral. To protect against being wiped out financially by inflation, they advised investing in "collectibles" like gold, other precious metals, diamonds, paintings, antiques, "things" with intrinsic value. These collectibles would maintain their value while securities and paper money would be nearly worthless in their predicted runaway inflation.

One famous story of the "gold bugs" was about the Weimar Republic in Germany in the 1920s when inflation was so rampant that the paper money, the German mark, was almost worthless. A man filled a wheelbarrow with German marks and left it outside a store while he went inside to make an inquiry. After a brief time in the store, he came out to find that someone had stolen the wheelbarrow and left the worthless bills.

Before my disability occurred, I had become interested in the "gold bug" literature and, as a consequence, purchased some gold coins. I began to look for articles about collectibles, especially gold.

Coincidentally, at this time, my feeling was that my life was going nowhere. I have recently read a description of my situation by Rabbi Robert A. Alper, calling it being "stuck in life." He compares being stuck in life with a rock climber stuck on a sheer rock cliff trying to find a way to move up. He says, "We know it is part of human nature to get stuck, to be afraid to move on, to worry that there is no way out of situations in which we find ourselves, situations that bring pain rather than happiness. We get stuck. And unless we constantly remind ourselves that there are solutions, our lives fill with despondency and frustration rather than joy and well-being."

Using my interest in gold to develop a business suddenly appealed to me as a possible means to get unstuck. Rather than purchase gold coins locally, I had done some research and found a reliable firm in a nearby state that did a mail-order business. In this way, the 7 percent sales tax was legally avoided, which was a considerable saving. The hype from the "gold bugs" was arousing a great deal of interest in gold from people who had never thought about buying it before. I discovered most of them were in the dark about how to purchase it.

I researched the gold business by requesting literature from every company that ran an advertisement selling gold.

Other sources were "gold bug" literature, newspaper, and magazine articles. This was exciting, and gradually, a plan evolved to establish a business as a consultant advising people why, where, and how to go about buying gold, usually coins, by mail order from out of state, conveniently at a fair price and a saving (no sales tax). This approach had proven very satisfactory and safe for me.

The business was called the Rainbow Investment Company, and I went so far as to register the name officially with the county. Business cards and literature were printed using my home as my office. I collected a list of about five out of state companies that had excellent reputations to be recommended to my clients during the in-depth consultation. At this time, the "gold bug" philosophy would be explained, the reason for purchasing gold and the mechanics of actually making a purchase.

The gold coin of choice was the South African Krugerrand which contained one troy ounce of gold. Just to show what was happening in the year before my retirement, I made purchases of

---

[1]   *Life Doesn't Get Any Better Than This,* Robert A. Alper, Triumph Books, Liguori, Missouri, 1996, pp. 106-113.

Krugerrands on August 2, 1979, at $304 per coin; on August 16 at $314; and on September 6 at $355. By January 1980, gold rose to $875 per ounce and then took a precipitous drop. Because of the lower price, it was being actively touted again.

My fee for a consultation and help making a purchase was $100. This was reasonable. As an example, if a gold coin sold for $300 and ten were purchased costing $3000, the sales tax saving of 7 percent would amount to $210, more than enough to pay for the advice and assistance. I actually had my first customer and was feeling good about the business until shortly thereafter a newspaper article in its financial section carried a story about one of the firms I was recommending but had never dealt with.

This firm had been in the precious-metal business for a long time and had a well-established reputation as a reliable company owned by a respected family. However, the article described how customers had sent in orders with checks but never received the gold or whatever they ordered. Telephone calls to the company were not returned. An investigation revealed that a member of the firm had absconded with the funds. The customers were the losers.

After reading about this firm, which was on my recommended list, I decided that I would be sticking my neck out and could get into serious trouble if one of my customers were cheated in this way. I decided the gold business was not for me and gave it up. It was fun for the short time that it lasted.

The next step in my search for an occupation was in the real estate field. My brother had a successful, active real estate business in Schroon Lake, and he assured me of a job if I obtained a salesperson license, which could be obtained by taking a course in the fall at nearby Adirondack Community College and then passing the licensing examination. This was done, and I obtained my license.

Before going to work as a real estate salesman, I did considerable soul searching. Was this the right type of work for me? In my field in the medical profession, there was satisfaction in seeing successful results in most patients quite quickly. In the real estate business, a salesperson spends a good deal of time with prospects with many failures before a sale is made. Could I be happy in this type of business? I realized it would be too frustrating, and my decision was no. Like in rock climbing, I had not yet found a foothold or anything to grasp to move up. I was still stuck.

Chapter 24

As 1980 drew to a close, my frustration and lack of success in improving my situation during the previous nine months were taking their toll. Blossom and others were very supportive, but it seemed that almost everything that I touched and tried fell through. The one bright spot was that my vision was returning to a useful level with corrective lenses in my glasses. Also, for the present time, we were managing to get by financially.

The home-office seemed like an encumbrance that no one was interested in. My practice had dissipated. My hopes for careers in the gold business and real estate had not proven realistic. It was a low point in my life.

To keep occupied, I spent many hours in the library and at home reading about retirement and then about aging and gerontology. Gradually, it dawned on me that perhaps I needed to utilize my vacant office in some way myself if no alternative materialized. I wasn't ready to contemplate removing all my valuable equipment and renting the space, since it was such an ideal setup for an otolaryngologist or allergist. There was no desire or temptation on my part to return to my previous medical practice because my vision would never be good enough.

However, my increasing familiarity with the problems of aging and retirement made me realize that in our community and nearby area, there was no professional practicing counseling of the aging, gerontological counseling. Could I fill this void? It seemed to me that my counseling experience in medicine, my knowledge of the problems of the aging, and some additional training would prepare me very adequately for a second career using my office space.

One of my good friends in the medical community here was a psychiatrist. I consulted her for advice regarding gerontological counseling, and she agreed that there was a need in the community for this service. Before recommending that I enter this field, she wanted to carry out a thorough psychiatric examination of me. This was to determine my suitability for this type of practice. I had no problem with this approach and gladly assented.

For more than two hours on each of two afternoons, she interviewed and questioned me about every aspect of my life. When the examination was over, the verdict was that I was very suitable for counseling, and she encouraged me to prepare to enter this field. Even more heartening was her invitation to attend her biweekly group counseling sessions for adults the next year as an observer. I shall ever be grateful for the generosity of her friendship, support, and professional courtesy.

With this encouragement, I enthusiastically began planning to train for a new career. It was not feasible for me to enter into a full-time academic program requiring several years. It was the beginning of 1981, and my plan was to prepare myself during the year and open a practice in 1982.

Since there was no chartered course to follow, I developed a program that included attending group-counseling classes twice a week, studying gerontological literature, attending a seminar on preretirement planning in New York City, attending the annual meeting of the Gerontological Society of America in Toronto, Canada, and going to several other conferences and seminars related to aging and retirement. In September 1981, I began a three-month part-time course in "Working with the Elderly" at the State University of New York (SUNY) in Albany. Professor Edmund Sherman, who taught the course, was also the author of a book on counseling the aging, which was a valuable adjunct to the course.

It was a busy and happy year for one who enjoys being a perpetual student, since being occupied kept me from dwelling on my problems. Also, Blossom traveled with me most of the time, which was enjoyable and good for both of us.

By the late fall of 1981, I was pleased with my progress academically, but my instincts told me that more practical personal experience was necessary to properly prepare myself for the practice of gerontological counseling. I began to inquire about internships in this field. Very little was available, but after much research, I found a program at the Hillsborough Community Health Center in Tampa, Florida, that offered the practical experience I was seeking. They accepted me for a ten-week program, and we happily chose to go to Florida during the winter months of January to March 1982.

It was quite an unusual experience both for the personnel of the center and for me. Most of their students had been at the college level. Those doing the teaching were at a master's level with a great deal of knowledge and experience. They had never had a sixty-eight-year-old physician as an intern, and they wondered about how we would relate. Fortunately, I have an inborn sensitivity that foresees problems of this nature. From the first day, I informed them that I was there to learn and would be accepting of their teaching and criticism. I asked to please be treated like they would any other intern. I was assigned to a preceptor, who was very capable and friendly, and we hit it off extremely well.

The program was not strictly structured but consisted in responding to calls requiring a social worker's intervention, working with nursing-home residents, and mostly group counseling at the center.

Many of the experiences were eye-openers and very instructive by introducing me to "hands on" contact with the seamy side of the aging process. For example, the center was notified by neighbors that a resident in their housing project was acting strangely. The apartment was in a low-cost housing project occupied mainly by the aging. We rang the doorbell and were admitted by an unkempt elderly woman into a house that was a mess. From what we could ascertain, she had no immediate relatives, lived in isolation, and, most likely, her only income was from Social Security. Her entire little apartment was stuffed with canned goods, including the refrigerator, closets, and living room. It was obvious she suffered from dementia (possibly Alzheimer's disease), but further studies would be needed to rule out other causes like malnutrition. She needed active intervention, and it was our duty to notify the proper authorities and services to take over her care. We did not do the follow-up care.

We visited nursing homes to observe and participate in programs designed to provide stimulation to the aging residents who otherwise spent their days not talking and looking blankly at the walls. One of the exciting experiences was to see many of them come to life when the old familiar songs were played by clapping their hands to keep time and singing along. Some even would get up and dance.

The experience was very valuable, and while limited in the amount of one-on-one counseling done in a private practice, I knew I was ready to return to Glens Falls and start to practice.

Blossom and I enjoyed our winter in Tampa. By this time, I could play golf, and we enjoyed playing on the courses there. We visited St. Petersburg and Sarasota and found the life around Sarasota very tempting. If we had not been stuck with our property in Glens Falls, it is very likely we would have moved to Sarasota.

Just to show how sheltered my life had been, in Tampa, I visited a "sex shop" for the first time. In the windows and front of the store, they showed black sexy lingerie, but once inside, you were directed to the back of the store where they had the most amazing collection of instruments and equipment to be used for personal sexual satisfaction and in relationships. I had heard about some of these things but never had any idea what was available and was being sold and used.

It was time to go home and go to work.

Chapter 25

My return to Glens Falls after the Florida experience began an exciting time for me. About two years after my forced retirement from my ear, nose, and throat and allergy practice resulting from disabling double vision, I was in good health with useful vision. My office was ready for use in my new career in counseling the aging. My approach would be gerontological, relating to the social, psychological, and economic problems of the aging. It was not geriatrics, which deals with the medical and surgical problems of this age group.

There was one exception. Since one of my main practice interests had been deafness and problems of the deaf and hard of hearing, I wanted to continue to utilize my expertise in this field. My equipment for testing hearing, which had not been used in two years, was state of the art, including a soundproof room. It occurred to me that it would be logical to combine audiology, a branch of science dealing with hearing, with counseling since many aging suffered from impaired hearing.

Fortunately, I was able to hire a very capable audiologist (a specialist in testing hearing) to work for me on a part-time basis, since audiology patients do not usually require immediate examinations. They can be scheduled by appointment. In an emergency, I could do basic testing.

To inform my medical colleagues and other sources of referrals for my new practice, I wrote them a letter detailing the scope of my services and the training that had prepared me in the field of counseling of the aging. In addition, a dignified advertisement was placed in *The Post-Star*. There was also an article in the paper about me and my return to a new practice.

In the beginning, there was a trickle of patients. My sights and enthusiasm focused on a much bigger goal than just a practice. Because in our area, as elsewhere, there was a lack of knowledge and understanding of aging and its associated problems as well as much misinformation, I resolved to start a one-man educational campaign to improve the situation. My approach was to prepare a talk, "Myths, Stereotypes, and the Aging," which I would present to any group seeking a speaker who would not charge for his services. In my approach to the subject, my motto was "Aging with optimism."

The following is the fact sheet to be used by the person introducing me to an audience:

Orel Friedman, M.D., recently opened his office at 591 Glen Street, Glens Falls, New York, for the practice of audiology and gerontological counseling.

Dr. Friedman's many years of experience with diseases of the ear will be concentrated in the field of audiology. The services he will provide are hearing testing and the diagnosis and nonsurgical treatment of children and adults with impaired hearing.

Gerontological counseling is a specialty dealing with the psychological, social, and adjustment problems of the aging. These problems can relate to marriage, widowhood, sexuality, mental and physical change, and the elderly and their families. Preretirement planning and retirement counseling are included in this field.

Dr. Friedman maintained an ear, nose, and throat practice for thirty years before closing his office two years ago. Since then, he has taken special training in counseling and working with the elderly. His goal is to dispel the myths and stereotypes which influence negative attitudes about aging and replace them with a positive approach to aging with optimism.

He is a graduate of the Glens Falls High School, Union College, and the Albany Medical College. His wife, Blossom, and he reside at 6 Arbor Drive in Glens Falls. They have three children and seven grandchildren. (Four more grandchildren were born after this time).

The defining moment in my rehabilitation and regaining my self-esteem occurred on the day I first presented my talk, "Myths,

Stereotypes, and the Aging." It was June 16, 1982, and my audience was the Kiwanis Club of Glens Falls at their weekly luncheon meeting in the Queensbury Hotel in Glens Falls. I worked very hard fine-tuning and rehearsing my talk, which included several jokes, as is my custom. One of my positive attributes is the ability to remember and tell jokes, which are not read but told from memory in a relaxed manner. In this way, the jokes have spontaneity and provide a welcome change of pace from the seriousness of the subject while emphasizing an important point that has just been made. I also reviewed all kinds of information, hopefully to be able to answer any question in the question period after the presentation. I was well prepared.

I wore my best suit and matching tie. I was nervous and just picked at the lunch. Happily, my talk and the jokes went over very well and were enthusiastically applauded. The compliments from the audience were sincere and heartwarming for me. I knew that my speaking debut had been a real success.

I was feeling very good about myself as I left the hotel and crossed the street in the direction of Crandall Library. It was still early afternoon on a beautiful spring day. I wanted to shout for joy, "I did it."

The first person I saw was one of our friends, a bright, friendly widow, who was sitting alone on a park bench enjoying the sunshine and fresh air. She most likely was there because of loneliness, hoping to find someone to talk to. We greeted each other, and she invited me to join her. I gladly accepted the invitation and sat down. It was a perfect situation because I was bursting with desire to tell someone about my wonderful experience at the Kiwanis luncheon, and she was sincerely interested in hearing about it.

She had no knowledge about my new career in gerontological counseling. After bringing her up to date about my activities, she asked me to read my talk, which was in a folder in my hand, to her. I did this and told her the jokes. She was very impressed because so much of my information was a revelation to her. We discussed the subject and problems of aging, and we sat there for quite a while. It was a most enjoyable experience for both of us. Ventilating my feelings was just what I needed. We parted, and I was anxious to go home and spill it all to Blossom. I told Blossom the good news, and she was happy because this was another step in the direction of a brighter future.

Chapter 26

As word spread about my practice and my interesting presentations, the second half of the year 1982 was a time of hope and increasing fulfillment. My patient load was gradually growing, and I knew that building a practice would take time. Speaking engagements brought me in contact with many interesting people such as retired teachers, various service clubs, and senior lunch groups. I was putting the subject of aging on the map in a positive manner.

Without my realization, Blossom saw me as a sixty-eight-year-old man on a mission who would be devoting my remaining years to a counseling practice. She knew how conscientious I was, and to do justice to my patients in counseling, our vacations and time away from Glens Falls would be short and limited. She knew what being tied down was like from my years of practice as an otolaryngologist who was devoted to his patients and profession. Then we were younger and were building a family life with children to support and educate. We had traveled and enjoyed ourselves, always knowing we had to get home fairly soon. At times, there were activities and family gatherings that had to be passed up, or Blossom would go alone because I couldn't get away. It was a necessary lifestyle in those years.

Also, winters in Glens Falls became harder to take as we grew older. Spending the previous winter in Tampa had been an enjoyable experience. If we had been able to sell our property in the early days of my retirement, we may well have chosen to move to Florida. Also, we had many family members living in Southern California. Blossom's sister, Razie, a divorcee, was living in a big, beautiful home in La Jolla, California, and wanted company. She invited us to spend the winter with her. I shrugged it off with the thought that we would go there for a couple of weeks, but Blossom had different ideas.

The thought of being tied down to a practice and spending our winters in cold, freezing Glens Falls became too much for her. One day, near the end of the year, she told me in her manner that experience had taught me meant there was no turning back, "I don't want to spend any more winters in Glens Falls."

I responded, "I can't do counseling on a part-time basis such as going away for months at a time." I admitted my dislike for the winters here. This was a crisis in our relationship, and my instincts told me to accede.

My answer was, "If you don't want to winter here, neither do I. Give me some time to close my office, and we'll go to California."

It was a bittersweet decision and a tribute to my good fortune in having a wife whose love, common sense, and wisdom had brought me much happiness. Her long-range vision certainly surpassed mine at the time. It was the proper decision as proven by the wonderful years and experiences of the rest of our lives together. This is well explained by the aphorism that recently came to my attention, "No man on his deathbed says, 'I did not spend enough time at the office.'"

On the surface, it appeared that the past two years spent studying gerontology and counseling and then starting a practice had been wasted. On the contrary, the knowledge acquired regarding the aging process enriched both our lives since Blossom had attended seminars, meetings, and shared my reading material. We discussed the knowledge we were acquiring. Decisions regarding our lifestyle and future were informed decisions based on a wealth of valuable information. We were on the right track.

Also, I had an identity, a gerontologist, and, in one way or another, continued to be involved in this field over the years as a lecturer, teacher, and resource person. The discovery that I was an excellent public speaker whose presentations were enhanced by an ability to tell jokes was a tremendous boost for my ego and self-esteem.

It goes back to the saying "Making lemonade out of a lemon." If not for my forced early retirement (lemon) and second career (the lemonade), the motivation to become a public speaker would not have existed.

In retrospect, the seeds were there from my youth. In high school and college, I participated in school plays, usually in minor parts. During my years of practice, I gave occasional talks to lay audiences on subjects like deafness but rarely spoke at professional scientific programs. As an officer at Temple Beth El, one of my duties was to make presentations at various functions.

In 1956, the Glens Falls High School Class of 1931 was celebrating our twenty-fifth year since graduation. It was tradition for this class to be invited to the graduation banquet for the current graduates. My classmates, to my surprise, asked me to make the customary speech for us at the banquet. This was an honor, and I was anxious to make a good impression. Many, many hours were spent preparing and rehearsing my presentation. When called upon to speak to an audience that filled the ballroom at the Queensbury Hotel, I was extremely nervous with a dry throat and pounding heart. However, all went very well, and I received many compliments.

A comparison of the anxiety of that experience to the pleasure and confidence with which I address an audience today has convinced me that public speakers are made and not born.

It would be ideal if every schoolchild were required to start elocution, the art of effective public speaking, in the earliest grades and continue to participate until graduation from high school. Competence in elocution should be required for graduation. This would greatly improve the grammar and sentence structure of the spoken English language of high-school graduates and those receiving advanced education. Some of the grammar and expressions used by professionals on radio and television are deplorable. It would also improve the students' writing skills if they were required to prepare the text of their oral presentations.

To return to our plans for the winter, by January 1983, my practice was closed, and we headed for La Jolla, California. There we had a wonderful time playing golf, sightseeing, and leisurely visiting with our many family members and a few friends in San Diego, La Costa (Carlsbad), Santa Monica, and Los Angeles.

The months in California had been quite carefree. With the advent of spring, it was time for the snowbirds to return to Glens Falls and face the reality of the unresolved problems we faced.

Chapter 27

Wintering in California had been a wonderful respite from our many unresolved problems. Now we had to face the fact that there was no longer any practice for an ear, nose, and throat specialist or allergist to take over and continue. It was expensive maintaining our home-office property without deriving any income from it. Despite continued effort, no interested buyer was found.

Unfortunately, the income from my disability insurance would soon terminate in accordance with the time limitations under the policy.

We were living on Social Security, income from IRAs and investments, and the soon-to-expire disability insurance. While not denying ourselves the necessities, we were living a more conservative financial lifestyle than before my retirement. This was in keeping with my approach to finances which I tried to teach our children using these truisms: "A fool and his money are soon parted." "Money is a good slave but a poor master." And from Charles Dickens's *David Copperfield,* where Mr. Micawber stated the following.

"My other piece of advice, Copperfield," said Mr. Micawber, *"is this: Annual income twenty pounds, annual expenditure nineteen, nineteen six, result happiness. Annual income twenty pounds, annual expenditure twenty pounds, ought and six, result misery."*

And finally, the statement that is framed and sits on my desk, "Man who gives his children a habit of industry provides for them better than giving them a stock of money," by George Ellis. I know that this last statement rubbed off on our children because they

---

1   *The Dickens Digest,* condensed by Mary Lou Aswell. Published by McGraw Hill Book Company, Inc., 1943, page 44.

are all hard workers. Also, they kid me and say, "We sure don't have any money," when I remind them of this truism.

Faced with a limited and fairly fixed income, I decided that the only way to have peace of mind financially would be to establish a budget. Budgeting by individuals is talked about considerably but is rarely practiced even though it is the keystone for good financial planning. Most people know what their income is, but few really know what their expenditures are unless they keep track by budgeting. It takes a full year to get an accurate picture of where and how your money is spent, and it requires discipline to keep track of even the little daily expenditures, which, in the course of time, can add up to a significant sum.

My personal system, which has served me well for almost twenty years, is relatively simple. Budgeting gave Blossom and me peace of mind in this time of financial uncertainty. After the first year, some surprising figures were found regarding some of our expenditures. After the first year, one can project what income is anticipated, and the expenses based on the previous year's findings should be manipulated not to exceed income. This may require painful decisions about lifestyle, but on the other hand, it curbs wasteful spending overlooked in the past, which can be eliminated without affecting your quality of life.

Budgeting has served me well in the years of my retirement, and eventually, I prepared a lecture, "Budgeting for the Retiree," which I presented to aging groups. However, there is considerable inertia when it comes to this type of planning, and I believe very few in my audiences followed my advice and instruction.

The wonderful thing about budgeting is the added pleasure that one can enjoy on a vacation knowing you can afford it and have included this expense in your budget. There are times when you go over your budget and invade your capital because of something you really want or must do. This is a calculated act, and if you are disciplined, you will not repeat it year after year. Sometimes you can compensate by cutting down on other discretionary spending. Living on a budget does not mean one has to be a miser.

We decided it was time to sell my office equipment and to advertise that it was for sale. An otolaryngologist, who had no equipment, was planning to open an office in a nearby city. A hospital in that city had offered to help finance his purchase of equipment since there was a shortage of practitioners in his specialty on their staff. He contacted me, and I negotiated with the hospital over the purchase price for everything in one package and made the sale. To be realistic, the sale of used equipment does not bring a price anywhere approaching its value even though it is high quality and in good condition, but the sale in one package was a stroke of luck and the best deal I could expect.

Since no purchaser for the building was on the horizon, I was trying to decide whether to rent my office space. A tenant would bring in rental income but also could foul up a sale if a prospective buyer came along. While vacillating over this decision, I was approached by an orthodontist practicing in Glens Falls who was seeking to rent new office space. He had heard about my empty office and was eager to rent part of it. It was ideal for him because the wiring for an X-ray machine was already in place, and the rooms were just the right size.

Since he was willing to accept a lease for one year at a time, I agreed to rent him the space he needed. There was still considerable office space that would be empty. It was late summer or fall 1983 by the time he moved in. Since the office was attached but a separate building, we both had our privacy.

It seemed like our fortunes were looking up. We kept busy playing golf, bridge, and square dancing. About one year after my retirement, we had joined the Merry Mohicans, a square-dancing club, and were greatly enjoying this delightful activity. We were meeting interesting people and making new friends. The colorful dresses worn by the women, the music, the caller and the intricate dance steps, and maneuvering with the three other couples in the set made the dancing fun and exciting as well as good exercise. Square dancing is organized nationally and internationally. During the winter spent in the Tampa area, we found a very compatible group of square dancers where we danced and made new friends.

In California, we were busy with family and friends and only danced a few times.

Also, it was great being retired, so we had the time and freedom to visit and be visited by our three married children and our grandchildren living in Rochester, New York City, and Cambridge, Massachusetts. We were settled into an enjoyable lifestyle with activities, family, and friends.

Our fortunes seemed to be improving with the sale of my office equipment and a tenant in my office. It was time to start thinking about where to spend the winter.

Chapter 28

Having spent the past two winters in Tampa, Florida and La Jolla, California, our desire was to spend the coming winter (starting January 1984) abroad in a warm climate. The Costa del Sol in Spain had been touted by travel magazines, newspaper advertisements, and friends as a very desirable place to winter.

Since one of my hobbies is planning trips and vacations, I began collecting brochures and information about the Costa del Sol.

There were several programs that fell within our budget for a winter vacation. The beauty of budgeting is that I had a clear idea regarding how much we could afford to spend on our winter arrangements. The value of the United States dollar was high and made vacations in Spain affordable. The American Association of Retired Persons (AARP) offered an attractive ten-week package of transportation to and housing in the hotel Castella de Santa Clara in Torremolinos on the Costa del Sol. An experienced representative of the AARP would be present there to help us with any questions or problems that might arise. We signed up early and were able to choose the location of our apartment in the hotel.

In the months before our departure, we studied travel guides, started to read Michener's *Iberia*, which I never finished, and found out about the many golf courses that would be available.

On all previous vacations, which had been short term or within the United States, my mail could be held or forwarded, and I handled our financial and other matters without difficulty. Going abroad for ten or more weeks presented a more difficult problem, which, at first, was worrisome, but as I began to reason, solving it became a challenge. This is the way I choose to handle stressful situations, looking upon them as a challenge and not a threat.

Little did I know at the time that solving this problem would eventually result in writing my booklet, *Worry Free Vacations Abroad*, published in 1987. The following is quoted from the first two paragraphs of the booklet:

An extended vacation abroad is just wishful thinking for most of us until retirement. When my dream first became a possibility, planning began by reading travel literature. Friends who had been abroad and travel agents were a valuable source of information.

I became euphoric thinking about exchanging the snow, cold, and darkness of a hometown winter for three months of warmth, sun, and new experiences in another country. The process of writing a check for a deposit suddenly jolted me back to earth. There was a lump in my stomach as I started to wonder about mail, paying bills, banking, income tax and closing our home. All of a sudden, the problems appeared overwhelming, and my mood changed to depression. Because of the obstacles should I take the easy way out and cancel my dream trip? Of course not!

I spent many hours working out the logistics and asked my accountant, Saul Silverstein, if he would handle our mail and financial affairs in our absence. He acceded, and all went well.

Prior to our departure, our son Victor and his wife, Nurit, presented us with a hard-cover notebook to use as a journal to record our experience in Spain. Blossom said to me, "You keep it." Although we had slides and photographs taken on all our trips, this was the first and, as it turned out, the only time I ever kept a journal of a vacation. To refresh my memory about Spain, I just reread the journal with great enjoyment and was amazed at how much had been forgotten.

Our vacation in Spain was another important transition in my life. The experience was very positive for both of us, but for me, it was proof that I could be completely relaxed and enjoy every day without any regrets about the circumstances that had forced me into an early and unexpected retirement.

Reading the journal now, I can appreciate the acting out of my changed attitude which had developed gradually since its low point more than three years previously. I had regained my self-confidence and self-esteem by realizing that my horizons had broadened from my previously more narrow focused life in medicine.

In Spain, I wrote several poems which were recorded in the journal. Otherwise, the poems may well have been lost.

My first entry in the journal dated 1/11/84, 11:25 PM, Torremolinos, Spain, describes our trip and first day in Spain. We arrived at our hotel in the morning and were checked in quickly. "Found our apartment clean, spacious, and facing the sea from a bluff and where the coastline makes a turn so the view is expansive and just gorgeous. Below is a large swimming pool, but it is not swimming weather, and a beautiful garden. The beach is quite narrow with a few hardy souls playing around in bathing suits in the warm noonday sun.

"About 2 PM we went for a stroll along the ocean walk where there is one restaurant after another—serving fish but meats as well. The prices and menus are posted outside, and dining is outside as well as inside with colorful tablecloths and decorations. What a selection, and the price is right." We picked out an attractive restaurant where we had an excellent swordfish dinner, with wine, delicious rolls, and fresh pineapple from South Africa for dessert. We were finished about 3:30 PM and decided to return to our hotel and get some sleep.

We had checked the beds on arrival, found them too soft for us, and asked for bed boards. "They hadn't gotten around to put them in, so we stopped at the desk to ask them again. They said *manana* [tomorrow], but we implored today without much hope of success.

"Inspired by the wine, sunshine, gorgeous surroundings, and something about a hotel room, we were in a lovemaking mood, and all was going great until two people, one male and one female, barged into our apartment using their own key to install the bed boards. Blossom put on a robe; I scurried for the bathroom and made it just in time. Then I got into the act a bit with a towel around me. It was good for a laugh for us, and I am sure it raised their appreciation for the AARP. I should give them the book *Sex and Sexuality in the Mature Years*. It was quite a first day."

My sleep pattern was off schedule, and about 4 AM of the next day, I was wide awake thinking about our lives and present lifestyle. I wrote this poem and called it "Aequanimitas," after the book written by the famous physician Sir William Osler.

Your retired life can be beautiful,
Your days and nights can be full,
Contentment and accomplishment can cull,
Fulfillment from the useless and dull.

Looking back, this poem truly represents my disengagement from the practice of medicine and gerontological counseling with no regrets.

Chapter 29

On our second day in Spain, we were taken on a bus tour of the area called Malaga Province, where there is everything from narrow, winding mountain roads to the coastal highway along the Mediterranean Sea. The towns, villages, and countryside are picturesque and full of buildings with interesting architecture. Everything looks very clean with flower gardens and landscaping. Along the roads are olive, orange, and lemon trees. There were also blossoming almond trees and pomegranate trees, which were not bearing fruit at the time.

We came down from the mountains at Marbella, a city noted as a gathering place for "high society."

In the evening, our AARP representative, Jane Bravery, gave us an orientation lecture about shopping, banking, laundry, restaurants, and tipping. She did not recommend renting a car. However, after our inconvenience and expense the next day taking a taxi to the Mijas Golf Course, about ten miles away, we decided that having our own car was essential if we were going to have a good time.

We spoke to Jane that evening and told her we wanted to rent a car. She offered to investigate rentals for us and, the next day, told us we could rent a Ford Fiesta with manual shift for $250 a month, including insurance. We told her to complete the arrangements. Jane has proven to be very pleasant, competent, and helpful.

We took a walk to explore the main shopping district of the city. Lladro is for sale everywhere.

Our apartment has a balcony with a view that inspired me to write this poem:

The Costa del Sol is what you see,
The sun is hot and bright as can be,
Its reflection glares in the shimmering sea,
For us, it seems the right place to be.

It is the custom in Spain to eat dinner late, starting at 8:30 or 9:00 PM. We tried it the first few nights but found it was too close to our bedtime. We were uncomfortable going to sleep on a full stomach and reverted to earlier dinners.

It is the morning of January 17, our sixth day in Spain, and we have a car. We decided to drive to Malaga, a few miles east of Torremolinos, and check out the golf course and the city, the local metropolis. We had just arrived at the clubhouse when a friendly woman started a conversation with us. This was the beginning of a most enjoyable day and a friendship that lasted throughout our stay in Spain. She was an American married to a native of Spain, who had lived and worked in the United States. They had retired to Spain and lived north of Malaga in a town called Casarabonela. Margaret, her husband, Tito, and a male friend were spending the day in Malaga.

The next day, I wrote a poem describing the wonderful experience.

MALAGA

We shall take the road to Malaga today,
While checking out the golf course on the way,
Met Margaret, to her a few words did say,
Leading to an afternoon so marvelously gay.

Coffee together on the patio facing the sea,
With husband, Tito, and a friend, they were three,
Quickly discovering how compatible we could be,
We drank and talked and laughed so happily.

They said, "Lunch with us at the Casa Pedro,"
This is where the natives, not the tourists, go,
On the way Malaga City, they did show,
It seems there isn't much they don't know.

The Sangria put us in a very relaxed mood,
To enjoy the gazpacho and paella, oh such food,
Endless conversation, jokes, until time did intrude,
We shared the check to avoid being rude.

Then off to El Corte Ingle's we drove,
The mammoth department store where to rove,
Everything from a pin to food for the stove,
Then, "Goodbye" to our friends, a treasure trove.

Shopping finished we drove back to our hotel,
Contentedly, the day had gone so very well,
With Americans, living in Spain, able to tell,
We are curious tourists, not living in a shell.

Ironically, we were so busy and enjoying ourselves that we never checked out the golf course. The next day, we went back and played it.

Torremolinos has its cool and dark days, and January 19 was such a day. I took a walk into town where I found people bundled up in hats and coats while others were walking around in shorts and sandals. The latter came here to escape from cold climates, and nothing will keep them from behaving like they are warm. The weather inspired me to write this poem:

CLOUDS OVER THE COAST

Today, Costa del Sol belies its name,
Lacking the hot sun that brings it fame,
Dark clouds over the beach, for shame,
Balcony cool, in the shadow its frame.

For only a second the sun breaks through,
As if it really knows what it must do,
To warm the chilly sweater laden few,
But then recedes, it can't get through.

Blossom told Jane that she wanted to join a dancing class where she could learn flamenco, Spanish dancing which has a great tradition. Jane made the arrangements, and Blossom attended the class throughout our stay. She enjoyed it immensely and, because of her natural dancing ability, became quite proficient.

Every Saturday evening, there was a bridge game for all the residents of the hotel. As couples came in, they sat down at or joined the next empty table, and the two pairs played together for the evening. We sat at an empty table and waited for the next couple to arrive. A short time later, a couple approached our table. As soon as I saw them, I said to the man, "I know you." He looked at me without recognition, and I said, "We interned together at the Beth El Hospital, my name is Orel Friedman." He then recognized me and told me his name, which I had forgotten. We had both been single as interns, and we introduced our wives, who were quite surprised listening to our conversation.

He practiced in Brooklyn and was still on the staff of the hospital. We talked briefly about ourselves and then had an enjoyable bridge game. After the game, we reminisced for a while and arranged to meet again soon, especially because he had so much information about former colleagues and the hospital that interested me.

January 22 was Super Bowl Sunday, but in Spain, it was just another day with no chance of getting the game on television.

Blossom likes to cook, and we enjoy eating on our balcony. Desirable fruits and vegetables are plentiful, and we like shopping in the supermarket. Freshly roasted chickens can be bought in stores nearby. Prices for food and restaurant meals are very reasonable.

Because of the strong dollar, retired Americans of limited means can live comfortably in Spain just on their Social Security. We were told that many American retirees were taking advantage of the low cost of living in Spain by making their permanent homes there.

Chapter 30

Our first twelve days in Spain have gone by rapidly. Happily for us, our accommodations, the Costa del Sol, the AARP support, and the people we have met have all lived up to expectations. We enjoy new experiences and adapt quickly to any environment that is strange to us.

Having a car gives us great mobility and opportunities to explore the area for golf courses, food, and other shopping and neighboring cities and towns. We have found people with whom to socialize and play bridge. We are looking forward to visiting some of Spain's interesting cities.

Two weeks had passed since we met Margaret and Tito, and we arranged to visit them. The following is quoted from my diary:

"It was a lovely day, and driving into the country is a never-ending experience of visual beauty and breathtaking scenes. Also there are some narrow, very winding roads. However, the small car is very maneuverable, and once one gets accustomed to the driving, there is no problem.

"On the way, we pass no end of orange groves, lemon groves, olive trees, houses perched on mountainsides, cultivated fields, freshly plowed fields, some livestock, flowers, dry river beds, and donkeys. In the towns and villages, there are narrow streets, people sitting in cafes, some hustling along but no great hustle, women wearing black dresses, and not many children as it is school time. One town looks like another. The mountains appear rocky and bare in the distance. The houses and villages on the mountainsides present a gorgeous picture.

"We arrived at our destination in quite good time. Their house is situated on a hilltop, and our hosts were waving to us as we approached from below. I don't think I am capable of describing their house, which is not finished yet but is a work in progress.

"In 1973, they bought the property, a small farmhouse with considerable land around it. It was once part of a large estate, and the farmhouse was like a temporary residence where the owners could come to work the land while maintaining their main residence in town. The Spanish are very family minded, and if they have a second home, they love to go back to their primary home where the action is to get together with family and friends.

"Margaret and Tito, working with four local laborers, have constructed a large, attractive home by adding on to and changing the original structure. They have six bedrooms, each with its own bath, and a magnificent master bedroom facing south with a gorgeous view. There is a large kitchen-dining room, the cabinets are wood, and the design is in squares, which is Castilian or a style of Northern Spain.

"They have plenty of water, which was the determining factor in their plans to build. All kinds of discarded materials are used. Tito has tremendous imagination and energy, and technically, he and his helpers can do everything necessary. He has a large old boiler that will be placed above a fireplace in a hidden manner to heat water. They are also planning to heat water using solar heat. Every room will have a fireplace, which will be built around some old funnel-shaped cement mixers he has acquired. The building stories go on and on.

"They also have land on which they grow wheat and garbanzo beans [chick peas] in alternate years.

"After the house tour and lunch, we drove around the town and then visited the olive-oil cooperative. The oil is in the pit, and we were introduced to the entire process of making olive oil. They sell the oil using a machine like a gasoline pump. The waste pits are used as fuel."

We drove through the town and were told that the street we were on had been named for General Franco, the Spanish dictator. Recently, the street was renamed by the new socialist government, thus obliterating Franco's name. There is considerable political "sanitation" going on in Spain.

After some tea and cake at our friends' home, we said our goodbyes. It had been a most enjoyable day, and the kind of day we relish where there is an opportunity to get close to the people in a foreign country.

Chapter 31

Several days later, we played the Torrequebrada Golf Course, the best of the courses we played in Spain. The course is long, difficult, and very hilly. We made a mistake in deciding to walk it rather than take a cart because, before long, the wind started to blow very hard, making walking difficult. It has a magnificent layout with lots of sand and water. There were fantastic views of the sea, which reminded me of the Torrey Pines course in San Diego, California. On the other side were the verdant mountains.

There were three tees for men, and even the white tees, which are the easiest, require long, straight shots over canyons and water on many holes. In the wind, my chances of getting across safely were too low, so I joined Blossom on the ladies tees from where I had a chance to get a satisfactory drive.

Even though the course was not crowded, it took five hours to play eighteen holes. On one hole, the wind was blowing so strongly we could not swing our clubs and had to pick up our balls. I was exhausted when the round was over, but Blossom said she enjoyed it. They should call the course Torquemada, in memory of the torturer, instead of Torrequebrada, because I felt like I had been tortured on a rack at the finish. I did not want to repeat this experience, but I was glad we tried it.

We played golf many times on about six different courses, and this contributed greatly to the pleasure of our stay.

Over the course of the next several weeks, we took trips to Grenada and the Alhambra, Cordoba, and Seville, all enjoyable and worthwhile. James Michener, in *Iberia,* ducked trying to describe famous places like the Alhambra because they had been adequately described elsewhere, and my approach is the same because I can't do justice to them. Our sister-in-law, Ruth Levitz,

joined us in Torremolinos for a while and visited Cordoba and
Seville with us. We also took a trip to Morocco and saw the Rock
of Gibraltar from the boat.

One of our unusual experiences was a day trip with our AARP
representative, Jane Bravery, on her day off. We asked her to pick
an interesting place to spend the day, and she suggested we go to
Cesares, a town in the mountains, and the drive there was along a
narrow, winding road with spectacular drop-offs. On the way, she
showed us cork trees. Many trees showed areas where the bark (the
cork) had been stripped from them.

Cesares is built on the side of a mountain and is famous for its
homes built in caves gouged out of the mountain. We saw one
store with several rooms inside the mountain. It is a unique and
worthwhile town to visit.

We had lunch in a little restaurant where we dined for two
and a half hours. No one rushes you. We ordered leg of lamb, but
they were able to serve only two portions. I had leg of goat for the
first time. It tasted very good.

The relaxed atmosphere and the wine led to an interesting
conversation during which Jane told us we were the nicest people
she had ever had under her care since she had been in the business.
It was pleasing to hear this from her, and we sincerely told her how
much we liked her and how well she was doing her job. It was
another wonderful day.

It seems that we had been on a "high" during our stay in Spain
with everything going well. However, on a Saturday, in preparation
for Blossom's birthday, I needed some cash. I always went to the
same bank to get a cash advance using my Visa card and felt like a
regular customer, but this time, when I presented my card, it was
rejected. They said they sent two telexes to the Glens Falls National
Bank but had no response, which was understandable since it was
6 AM at home. Then I submitted my MasterCard and received the
reply "no good." I knew I had sufficient funds in my bank, and I
had a terrible letdown feeling. One minute, the bank official was
friendly and happy to see me, and after the rejections, he acted in

a very cold and impersonal manner toward me, although he had previously carried out numerous transactions for me in a congenial manner.

Fortunately, I always carry a traveler's check for such an emergency and was able to obtain the needed cash. On the following Monday, I tried my Visa card again and obtained the cash advance without any difficulty. I believe it had something to do with communications on the weekend. This was a traumatic experience for me because it is in my nature to make the proper financial arrangements when I am at home or away.

March 11 was Blossom's birthday, and we planned to celebrate by having a dinner party with several of our friends at our favorite restaurant, The Portofino, in Fuengirola, a nearby town. Their specialty is lamb, and you must make a reservation and put in your order at least one day in advance or they won't serve it to you. When your party is seated, the dinner is ready. It was a superb dinner of lamb, roasted potatoes, string beans, french fried onions, and tasty wine. I wrote a poem for the occasion and read it at the party.

HAPPY BIRTHDAY, BLOSSOM

Happy Birthday, Blossom, wife ideal,
The love, all who know you feel,
Your beauty, charm, and wisdom reveal,
A personality with irresistible appeal.

Superior person with the common touch,
Things and position do not matter much,
Empathy for the disadvantaged and others such,
Leaned on by many as a strong crutch.

Beloved Bubbe of grandchildren, all eight
Worship her as the greatest of the great,
How lucky for her it was her fate,
That I chose her for my mate.

I knew the last two lines would get a rise out of her and prepared two more endings for the poem to quickly get back in her good graces as follows:

or

How lucky for me it was my fate,
That she chose me for her mate.

or

How lucky for us it was our fate,
To choose each other for our mate.

At that time, we had eight grandchildren and, later on, were blessed with three more. What the ending of the poem really says is, "The best thing that ever happened to me was marrying Blossom." It was a great birthday party.

On March 15, we flew to Madrid for a four-day visit. Spain is not real warm in the winter, and since Madrid is further north than Torremolinos, we waited until the end of our stay to visit there hoping it would be warm. We visited the Royal Palace, which was not used as a residence by Juan Carlos, but is used for state functions, especially the beautiful banquet hall which can seat 150 diners.

It contains the world's greatest collection of centuries-old tapestries. There are paintings by the masters, furniture, precious metal objects, china, clocks, religious garments, and ceramics in the famous collection. The chandeliers and rugs are magnificent, and there is a museum of musical instruments.

The next day was cold and drizzly, but we took our planned side trip to Toledo. It was an ancient capital of Spain and a center of Jewish life and culture in the past.

We spent most of the next day at the Prado. It has a magnificent collection with many Goyas, El Grecos, Rubens, Titians, and Velazquezes. We thoroughly enjoyed it, but the day was hard on our backs and feet.

At the Prado, we had one of those "small world" experiences. My secretary for many years, Joyce Harrison, has a son, Andrew, who is a teacher at a private school in Connecticut. During vacation break, he was touring Europe with a group of his students, and we met in the museum. He recognized us and said hello. We chatted only briefly because he had to keep moving with his group.

In the evening, we went on a tour that took us to dinner and then a night club and a flamenco performance. The night club was deafening disco and rock, and the flamenco was terrible. We had looked forward to a big night on the town for our last one in Madrid, but it was very disappointing.

The following day, we returned to Torremolinos.

Chapter 32

After returning to Torremolinos, only three days were left before our departure for home. We played golf, lunched with friends, and had a delightful last-minute surprise visit from Margaret and Tito. They were in the area with their friend Dick because they were helping him find an apartment nearby. This is the entry I made in my journal after the visit.

"They had eaten late, and Tito brought a bottle of champagne, so we decided to stay in the apartment. Blossom brought out olives, cheese, and breadsticks. After talking for quite a while, we had rice pudding, coffee, and cake. It worked out beautifully. We had a marvelous discussion—Margaret knows her history, and both are informed about so many subjects. I warmed them up with some of my jokes and even read them some of my poetry. They liked the poem I wrote about them. They left about 12:30 AM in a pouring rain."

Regretfully, we never saw them again.

March 20 was another rainy day and a good day for packing and reading. I read most of the book *Vital Maturity*, published in 1979 by the late Morton Puner. He was the brother of Sherley Plasse, our daughter Barbara's mother-in-law. It is an excellent book, and he has a very comprehensive grasp of the subject of aging. We knew him well.

The wonderful thing about a journal is that it captures your thoughts at the time you are thinking them and not some time later in reflection. This is my entry on our last day in Spain.

"March 21, 1984—6:30 AM. I woke up early—our call was for 7 AM. Blossom is sleeping soundly. I have already done my exercises.

"On this morning of departure, which has arrived with unbelievable suddenness, I can say it has been an excellent winter for us in Spain. We had a good time, learned and saw a great deal, and, above all, made friends and enjoyed companionship. At this time, I think we have a right to feel very good about ourselves. Jane Bravery, our AARP representative, repeated to us that we were the most outstanding couple she had ever had in her years in this field. She always looked forward to our critique of trips, places, and hotels and valued our opinion.

"Blossom has a charming, positive personality and great curiosity, and she attracts people and friends so we don't lack for companionship to supplement our own relationship. Although we enjoy being together, our personalities demand wider expression. All in all, life here has been good to us, and we are anxious to say hello to family, friends, and soon grandchild no. 9.

"Adios Spain!"

However, the saga hasn't ended. First, I have to get something off my chest about Iberia, the Spanish National Airline, which had treated us very badly in South America in 1968. We were with a tour and arrived at the airport in Buenos Aires, Argentina, early in the morning for a relatively short flight to Santiago, Chile. We were told at the airport that our flight would be delayed for a considerable time. There were flights on other airlines that could have accommodated us and taken us without delay, but Iberia refused to allow us to exchange our tickets. As a result, we spent about twelve hours waiting in the airport before Iberia flew us to Santiago. We wasted a full day of our tour and felt like we had been held hostage. I said I would not fly on Iberia again, but when we signed up for the AARP trip, we were forced to fly Iberia.

What ensued next is described in detail in my journal entry dated March 22, 1984, which I have edited slightly.

"If you have time fly, especially if you are flying Iberia, you can expect anything. What this airline is missing is communication-they are so secretive we could be on a mission for the CIA or KGB.

"After the usual checking in and waiting for our flight, Blossom and I had a nice chat with Jane Bravery, our leader. After take off and a brief flight, we landed at the Malaga Airport and were herded off the airplane to a waiting room while it was being refueled.

Without any explanation, the passengers were herded into another waiting room. Then we were moved back to the first waiting room. In the group were some "pushers," who have to be first even though there are seats and room for everybody. After about two hours of purposeless movement, we took off for New York City's [NYC] Kennedy Airport.

"All seemed to be going well, though the chicken for lunch was very greasy. Then we settled back for a James Bond movie, *Never Say Never*, which killed a couple of hours and a lot more people, including attractive girls. Then we filled out the customs declaration and settled back to do some reading with the feeling that we would land at Kennedy on schedule.

"We arrived on time over NYC and appeared to be circling for about thirty minutes. No information was forthcoming from the 'holy of holiest,' the pilot's cabin. Finally, word came over the loudspeaker, 'Because of weather conditions, we can't land and are going on to Montreal.' So, after a bit longer than the twenty-five minutes they said the trip would take, we landed at the Mirabel International Airport and sat on the strip. Still no information—are we disembarking, etc.? No word.

"For Blossom and me, disembarking in Montreal would have been OK. We could rent a car and drive home. It was only 4:30 PM.

"Finally, the word came—we are going to refuel—everyone stay on the plane, but NO SMOKING. By this time, it appeared that most of us would miss connecting flights, and there was no way we could communicate this problem to anxious families and people driving long distances to pick us up. Also, by this time, the bathrooms were getting pretty messy. Finally, the word came that we were taking off for New York City.

"It was still light when we headed south. After about twenty minutes, we encountered an electrical storm, and apparently, the left side of the plane was struck by lightning. We saw the flash on the other side, but there was no shock, loss of lights, or any disturbance. People on the other side said they saw the plane hit. It soon was apparent that we were flying low and saw the sun setting on our left. There was no sign of the Adirondacks, Albany, or lower New York State. I deduced that we were heading north towards Montreal, but not a word of information was given us until we landed safely at Mirabel International Airport in the middle of nowhere surrounded by all the emergency equipment for handling a crash landing.

"We sat in the plane awaiting some information. Finally, they said we would disembark and wait near carousel no. 3 while the Canadians on the plane would have to go through customs. So we got off and waited, not knowing what would come next. Blossom called our daughter Barbara and explained our delay. There was a big line for two phones for four hundred people, so the call was brief. Between 6:30 and 7:00 PM, the word came that we would go to the hotel and have dinner at 8:30 PM.

"So off went the four hundred of us—'Their's not to seek reply; their's but to do or why?' We only had our carry-on luggage as we were taken through a winding course and finally arrived at the hotel Le Chateau de l'Aeroport, a modern hotel. They handed out registration slips—two people had to check in the 'four hundred'— it took hours, and it was steaming hot in the lobby. The 'pushers' were doing business as usual.

"Around 9 PM, we got into our room, washed up, and went down, and had a special meal, tomato juice, beef stew, etc., that they set up in the ballroom and conference rooms for this large crowd. Our room is lovely and next door to the Scolas—our neighbors at the Castilla in Spain. We ate with them and four high-school kids, three girls and a boy, returning from a couple of weeks in Spain, Portugal, and Morocco as part of a group on vacation. From the conversation with them, it seems their trip was not much of a learning experience—sunning on the beach was the most enjoyable part according to one of them.

"We called our daughter Barbara, but she was asleep. We spoke to her husband, Terry, who told us it is foggy in New York City, but the weather is not bad. We deduced that being stacked up over Kennedy Airport may have threatened a shortage of gasoline, and we went to Montreal to refuel? Anyhow, we go back to Kennedy tomorrow. Now for some sleep.

"I was awake at 6:30 AM, although our awakening call was for 7 AM. I'll do my exercises. Blossom is still sleeping. She has a cold and a blocked ear.

"No luggage came off the plane, so I guess the Montreal people will also have to go back. They never went through customs. Our plans are to stay in New York City overnight and see our family.

"I must remark how great our aging companions are. The vast majority, and I assume that some of the people were in their late eighties, took this nerve-wracking, fatiguing day with strength, courage, and relatively good spirits. We are a very resilient group and excellent travelers. There was plenty of normal griping and always the few 'pushers' and inconsiderate people. All in all, we can be proud of our aging as people and travelers."

Our saga continues a little longer, with apologies to Alfred Lord Tennyson:

IBERIA

Theirs not to seek reply,
When with Iberia they fly,
In the dark skies don't try,
So flew the "four hundred."

"March 25, 1984. The previous entry was on March 22, in Montreal, our day of departure. That morning, we dressed and had a continental breakfast which we enjoyed with three other couples.

"It appears that the sequence of events the day before were as follows: (1) stacked up over Kennedy until our gasoline was becoming low, cause of stacking not definite, probably just very heavy traffic; (2) need to fly to Montreal to refuel; (3) on way back to Kennedy struck by lightning which knocked out the hydraulic system on (?) one or both wings; (4) pilot had a crippled plane, so he turned around and flew slowly at a low altitude to Mirabel Airport in Montreal very skillfully (although a little bumpily) under the circumstances and avoided a possible tragedy;(5) after a chance to evaluate the situation, it was decided that the plane could be repaired overnight, and we would fly to Kennedy Airport in the morning, which we did.

The arrival in Kennedy was smooth, and we landed without any delay. The luggage came off the plane in record time—we went through customs, paid a little duty, rented a car, and drove to Barbara's apartment house in New York City where we checked our car in the basement garage.

"We then took the elevator, and as we entered it, a little boy said, 'I know you.' It was our grandson Eitan, with their housekeeper. He was so cute.

"Anyhow, dinner tonight at Moshe Pekins Restaurant [Kosher Chinese] with Barbara and Terry, their sons, and Terry's parents, Sherley and Herman Plasse. It was a nice reception.

"Then up early in the AM and off to Glens Falls—quite a bit of snow on the ground. Found all OK at home. It is good to be here.

"Rhoda and George Forrest invited us to dinner. We are so lucky to have family and friends to say goodbye and greet us on our return.

"On a basis of 1 to 10, I would rate our Spanish experience as a 9.

"We had called Victor from New York City, and he informed us that all was OK, but Nurit was still waiting to deliver. They are living in the Cambridge, Massachusetts, area while he attends the Harvard Graduate School of Education.

"I wish to thank Nurit and Victor for giving me the journal and motivating me to keep this record."

Chapter 33

The joy of returning home after an idyllic vacation was spoiled by some bad news we received shortly before our departure from Spain. The following explains what happened.

I described previously that in the fall of 1982, after my decision to retire from gerontological counseling, I had the good fortune to sell my equipment and rent half of my office space to an endodontist.

About six months after renting to the dentist, a rheumatologist coming to Glens Falls to open a practice approached me about renting the other half of my office to him. It was perfect for him, and we agreed on a short-term lease like the one given my first tenant.

As a result, our financial situation had improved considerably, and we were more relaxed about selling our property since we loved our home, which was a most comfortable and spacious gathering place for all our children and grandchildren.

The bad news we received in Spain was that our endodontist had given the three months' notice that he was leaving the office and was moving to another city. It was disappointing and a letdown just when everything seemed to be going well. After he moved, no one sought to rent the office space.

I kept busy with speaking engagements during the spring, summer, and fall because I had a message promoting aging with optimism. As I remarked previously, local organizations were always seeking interesting speakers who did not charge for their services.

It was an exciting time as grandparents since we were free to visit our children's families who were living in New York, Rochester, and the Boston area. Also, they visited us often, and we had great times in our home, in Schroon Lake with our Friedman family at their camp on the east side of the lake, and with the Busmans in Bolton Landing.

We had a good time playing golf at the country club and in cities where we had golfing friends.

During the summer, I read an article in the *B'nai B'rith International Magazine* describing a three-month volunteer program for retirees in Israel sponsored by B'nai B'rith for the first time the previous winter. B'nai B'rith is an international Jewish service organization to which I belonged. Since we planned on going away for the winter, doing volunteer work in Israel appealed to us. Featured in the article was the story of a romance that developed between two of the volunteers who then married and were living in Pittsfield, Massachusetts, the wife's hometown.

Our very dear friends and golfing companions, Betty and Howard Braun, lived in Pittsfield. I called them and asked them if they knew the couple, and it turned out they were good friends. They also told us that the couple were very enthusiastic about their experience on the program and highly recommended it. The Brauns told us they could arrange for us to visit this couple if we came to Pittsfield, and we set a date for the visit.

Howie and Betty took us to the newlyweds' home, and we found them very gracious and enthusiastic about their experience. We decided that the program was worth pursuing and wrote to B'nai B'rith for their information packet.

After reviewing all the information and the costs, we decided that it would be an interesting, worthwhile, and affordable way to spend the winter in a hotel in Netanya, Israel. This was only about fifteen miles from Zichron Yaakov, the home of the parents and many family members of our Israeli daughter-in-law, Nurit. It was also close to Israel's only golf course in Caesarea. Israel is a Mediterranean country, and the weather in the winter is much like Spain. Winter is also the rainy season. We would not see Victor, Nurit, and their children, however, because they were living in the United States while he was studying for his doctorate in education at Harvard University.

We were accepted into the program and received all the information for our departure near the end of December on a charter flight from New York's Kennedy Airport. Blossom and I were very excited about the experience we faced.

The program began in December and finished in March and was well conceived. There were one hundred participants divided into two groups of fifty who stayed in two different hotels near each other and carried out most of our activities as independent units guided by a mature professional leader (called in Hebrew as our *madrycha*).

When we arrived at Ben Gurion Airport in Israel, we received an enthusiastic welcome organized by B'nai B'rith leaders and officials in Israel and the minister of information for the Begin Government, Morton Dolinsky. Mort, as we came to know him, was the cousin of Sherley Plasse, our daughter Barbara's mother-in-law. He had immigrated to Israel from the United States many years previously, and although we had never met him, we were very friendly with his sister, Shirley Kalb, who had alerted him that we were in the group. We were quite surprised when this top official, whom we had heard about but never met, sought us out and greeted us personally. This was the beginning of a friendship that lasted many years until his death.

In the other group of fifty volunteers was Fay Simkin, from Pittsfield, Massachusetts, whom we had met previously through our mutual friends, Betty and Howard Braun. Fay was the widow of Dr. Stanley Simkin, who was a student at the Albany Medical College when I was there.

Weary from our trip and happy to be in Israel, we were taken by bus to our hotel, the Sironit, in the seaside city of Netanya. There we received another "very important person" (VIP) welcome and banquet. It was well meaning and a wonderful beginning, but our fatigue began to show, and I felt I was being "killed with kindness." When the party was over, we "hit the sack" and had no trouble sleeping.

Chapter 34

Our next few days were spent in orientation, choosing our work assignments, and familiarizing ourselves with Netanya, a picturesque resort city on the Mediterranean Sea, with the most attractive seaside promenade in Israel. Our program was planned during the winter season to provide occupancy for the resort hotels during their slow season. The winter is also the rainy season, when the temperature can drop to 50 degrees Fahrenheit or go up to 70 degrees or higher. I remember playing golf on New Year's Day in my shirtsleeves. The sea is usually too cool for swimming during the winter months.

An article I wrote for a weekly newspaper in Albany, New York, *The Jewish World*, with the heading "Elderly Volunteer Programs in Israel Called Enriching," which appeared on August 11, 1988, best describes the experience and is quoted below:

Five years ago, 50 Jewish American volunteers aged 50 and over pioneered a work study program in Israel. This has to be one of the leading success stories of the decade-because five years later almost 500 volunteers participated in a similar program. My wife, Blossom, and I served as volunteers four years ago and again this past winter. We have observed this phenomenal growth. The first contingent called Active Retirees in Israel (the acronym ARI means lion in Hebrew) was sponsored by B'nai B'rith in cooperation with the World Zionist Organization Department of Aliyah (immigration) in Israel. They lived in a comfortable seaside hotel in the lovely Mediterranean resort city of Netanya.

Work, Study, Play

The ARI volunteers worked five mornings each week in hospitals, schools, Jewish National Fund forests, nursing homes and facilities for the handicapped. Part of most afternoons during the week were spent in Hebrew classes. Several evenings a week were devoted to lectures, discussions, social and cultural events. Among the areas visited in Israel were Jerusalem, the Negev, the Golan and the Galilee. This program has been a winner because of its sound concept-that many Jewish American retirees would jump at the chance to prove they are useful, needed and contributing members of society within the framework of an Israel experience.

Hadassah Involved

In the second year of the project Hadassah was invited to sponsor a group in order to broaden the base of volunteers. Four years ago we went with B'nai B'rith and this past winter with Hadassah in their WIN (Winter In Netanya) program.

Although we have been to Israel many times since our first visit in 1962, ARI and WIN have been different and more enriching experiences. No longer were we tourists staying in luxury hotels, seeing the wonderful showplaces but having little contact with the people. This time our activities brought us in contact with the everyday life of the Israelis.

Because of my interest in gerontology I worked as a volunteer in an old age and nursing home. Fortunately I had learned Yiddish (a language from Eastern Europe) growing up in Glens Falls because that was the best way for me to communicate with residents in the home originally from Eastern Europe. Blossom has worked in several areas: a botanical garden, as an English language tutor, preparing craft kits for the handicapped and in a senior citizen center. Four years ago we enjoyed doing conservation work in the Jewish National Forest.

The enthusiasm of the volunteers was more than matched by the positive feedback and show of appreciation we received from the Israelis. It is important to realize that we did not take a job away from anyone. We filled a void and carried out essential tasks that otherwise would not be done because of a lack of finances and other volunteers.

We were guests in Israeli homes and ate more cake on these visits than was good for us. Netanya has a large English speaking community and a very active Association of Americans and Canadians in Israel

(AACI) chapter. We were invited to join in their activities. Our contacts were with children, adults, the aging, workers and merchants. We were treated like VIPs (very important people).

It was amazing how rapidly our group, which had joined together as strangers, became a family in the course of a few weeks. Many singles participate in these programs because they are assured of companionship, and no one is left out. Each group of 50 or less has its own madrichya (leader), a full time Israeli "mother hen" to look after her brood. Olana Ostroff, our madrichya four years ago, and Jackie Schwartz, our leader this past winter, are unbelievably capable, caring and loveable. They were always there to insure our welfare in case of illness and to resolve the many problems that were bound to arise. Four years ago ARI had the unique experience of being in Netanya when 400 Ethiopian Jews were unexpectedly brought to an empty hotel near ours as a result of "Operation Moses." The Israelis had no way to prepare for this sudden great influx, and the cultural shock on the part of the Ethiopians and the language barrier made for very trying times for everybody. That we were available as volunteers to help out was an experience and privilege we'll never forget.

Our Ari experience led to the development of a close friendship with a couple in Netanya, Rebecca and Meyer Passow. He was an American-born rabbi who had moved to Israel to teach at Bar Illan University, from which he had recently retired. She was from Montreal originally, and it was a second marriage for both of them. We were invited to their home through the Ari home hospitality program, and we fell in love with each other. Meyer was a brilliant scholar and a wonderful conversationalist with a great sense of humor. When we started swapping jokes, we knew we were meant for each other. He had a magnificent library, and often, when we would discuss a subject or a famous individual, he would show me an autographed copy of the person's book. In Netanya, there was an excellent library of books in the English language, which he helped support by giving a series of lectures every year. We attended several of his lectures on a variety of subjects relating to the Jewish people, and they were excellent. Rebecca was a very gracious hostess.

There were a few people whose friendship and relationship have highlighted and influenced my intellectual and spiritual growth in the important years of my retirement, and Meyer was one of them. We visited them as often as we could during the six years until his death in 1990. He was important in my life.

Another meaningful experience was volunteering to help orient the Ethiopians who arrived in Israel unexpectedly on Operation Moses, when thousands of them were flown out of camps in Sudan as an emergency to prevent their slaughter. Israel had to find housing, social workers, and medical personnel overnight to service these newcomers, whom they welcomed with open arms. Although it was winter, they had to house several hundred refugees in a summer hotel with no heat. The cultural shock and language barrier compounded the problems.

The local community held a clothing drive when they heard the Ethiopians were coming, and they had outfitted the newcomers with a style of clothing that was unfamiliar to them and needed alterations to fit properly. We were asked to come and assist the limited staff and also bring needles and thread.

People were sitting on the floor in the hallways since there was nothing for them to do. Blossom found two brothers, probably twins, who had been given sneakers, but they had no idea how to wear them. One had two left sneakers and the other two right ones. She changed them so they had correct pairs and showed them how to lace and tie them. The boys got a big kick out of the procedure and showed their appreciation with a big laugh. Our group helped with clothes and did alterations.

What was fortunate for the staff who could not speak Amharic, the Ethiopian language, was the presence in a school in Netanya of several Ethiopian youths who were able to act as translators for the Hebrew-speaking Israelis.

The newcomers did not know what vacuum cleaners were or the purpose of plugs in the bathtubs. We showed them how to use appliances, and they were surprised and grateful.

Our friend, Fay Simkin, was a nurse, and she and I visited every room to check out those lying in bed to determine if they were ill. All the new arrivals had been examined medically before coming to Netanya, and the seriously ill ones had been hospitalized. However, we found that many had colds and other illnesses. We listed those we felt should be seen by a physician. There was one infant who appeared seriously ill, and we recommended immediate hospitalization. This was carried out, and we found out later that the infant had died of tuberculous meningitis.

We followed the newcomers over a period of several weeks. The men, children, and some women very quickly began to receive instruction in the Hebrew language. It was amazing how quickly the children picked up the language and played with Israeli children. Most of the adult women had babies and children to look after and could not attend Hebrew-language classes or go downtown to get oriented to life in the community. A dynamic group of Netanya women, especially those who had come from South Africa, quickly recognized this problem. They held fund-raising events and made enough money to set up a modern nursery for the infants and a nursery school for the preschoolers. This freed up the mothers to attend Hebrew classes and go into town. It was a wonderful accomplishment.

We had the opportunity to observe and appreciate the splendid job of absorption under the most trying circumstances that Israel had been doing since its founding to carry out its mission as a homeland for all Jews. It was a privilege for us to be able to help.

I elected to work in an old-age and nursing home. The director was an American who had migrated to Israel. He was very friendly and competent, and I enjoyed my experience working with him. However, my position was that of a volunteer helping out with tasks that improved the quality of life of the residents, like taking them out in wheelchairs to sit in the sun or playing games with them. The staff did not have time for many of these tasks. I also worked in the dementia section. One evidence of the advanced planning of the unit was a large outdoor fenced-in area where the residents could safely wander and walk. Some of them spent hours just doing that, and this was a great asset.

I found that the services provided by the state of Israel for their aging was caring and competent, considering the limited resources of the country. There was no charge for the care in this governmental institution, even though some of the residents had migrated to Israel in their later years and never worked or contributed to the health system. I greatly enjoyed working there during both of my winters as a volunteer.

On the Ari program, we spent one or two days a week doing conservation work in the Kadima Forest outside of Netanya. This was work that had been neglected because of lack of funds and manpower. Under the supervision of a trained Israeli, we cleared brush and trimmed and removed small trees using loppers and saws. We had a fun time working in the woods. One of the bonuses was working at times near an orange grove where we were given oranges, and once near a strawberry patch where we were given fresh strawberries.

We had great trips, educational programs, and social experiences on these volunteer programs which proved to be most enjoyable and worthwhile. Needless to say, we became a family of fifty people.

When the program was over, we returned to the United States with the satisfaction of having served others but had received more from the Israelis than we had given.

Chapter 35

Returning home from Israel was again a bittersweet experience comparable to what happened when we returned from Spain the year before. After enjoying our ARI program so much, we returned to Glens Falls knowing that our remaining office tenant had given notice that he was leaving the city. This meant that the income we depended on from our office space was gone.

After getting settled at home, we had a stroke of fortune when a friend referred a prospective buyer of our property to us. We sold the property, and it was a good deal for both parties. We had to close early enough for the family moving in to get settled before school started. Just as soon as the contract was signed, we hired our good friend and neighbor, Irene Fitzgerald, owner of Fitzgerald Realty to find us a home.

We wanted to downsize, and we felt that at our age living on one floor would be most efficient, practical, and comfortable. Also looking ahead to possible illness and disability, the avoidance of stairs made sense. I had told Blossom that living in an apartment without the responsibility of caring for a house suited me just fine. She said she wanted a house, lawn, and garden and would be responsible for taking care of the grounds, so I acceded to her wishes, and we decided to look for a ranch house.

I liked the idea of living in Glens Falls and being able to walk downtown, but we could not find anything suitable for us in the city. After looking at several homes in Queensbury, we found the home at 7 Sweetbriar Lane in Queensbury desirable and suitable. We purchased it since we could take possession in time for us to move from our old home. We had a busy summer preparing to move.

Our home and office on Glen and Arbor Drive had been on the market for five years before we finally sold it. We were happy to divest ourselves of this attractive property which had become a financial burden to us.

Our new home was a good choice, but it was not air-conditioned, and we moved in during a very hot spell in August. We immediately obtained two window air-conditioners, which helped somewhat. We had a lawn in front and in back, and the back of our property was a wooded area. The entire back of the property was enclosed by a chain-linked fence. The house had a full basement which contained the laundry, and it could be entered from the rear by a Bilco door, which made it easy to move things in and out of the basement without having to go through the house. Our predecessor in the home had built an airplane in sections in the basement and had installed this door so he could remove the airplane in sections. According to the seller, he actually flew the airplane. We also had a two-car garage.

Since we had no mortgage on our old property and were downsizing, we found ourselves with cash to invest to increase our income somewhat. Also, we felt comfortable deciding to spend six weeks of the next winter in Australia and New Zealand, which would have been too expensive for our budget before we sold the property. We already knew about the AARP program to this area from their catalogs and decided this would be the way to go. We signed up for the regular three-week program and picked electives for three additional weeks. We also planned a stay in Hawaii for a few days to break up our return trip to Southern California where we planned to stay about six more weeks before returning to Glens Falls.

During the previous year, Blossom's younger sister, Adelle Frank, had been diagnosed with breast cancer and was receiving therapy. The feeling was that her brothers and sisters and their spouses should all get together around Thanksgiving. Sid and Bert Levitz hosted a special dinner just for us in their home in the La Costa Golf Course Development. Everyone came from Florida, Arizona, and Glens Falls, but unfortunately, Blossom's older sister, Razie, was hospitalized in San Diego a few days before the affair and could not attend. Although this dampened our pleasure somewhat, we had a real good time together at a great dinner party. Also, since we were all in the area, we were able to visit Razie in the hospital. This was good for her morale, because she was diagnosed with lung cancer.

Our return home after this important family affair was marred by a bizarre incident. Thinking ahead to our trip to Australia, we had decided to break up the lengthy trip by spending a few days with our friends Shirley and Edgar Miller, who were former Glens Falls residents. Since our plane would be leaving from San Francisco, this was an opportunity to accept their longstanding invitation to visit them in Redwood City, which was near San Francisco. Since, on our return from Australia, we would be staying in La Costa, in Southern California, it made sense to take our golf clubs and other clothing with us at Thanksgiving time and leave them to be available on our return. We returned home with one large brand-new suitcase containing the belongings of both of us.

When we arrived at our eastern destination, the airport at Albany, New York, our suitcase did not arrive with us. We reported this to Baggage Claim, and being seasoned travelers, we knew they would follow through when they said the suitcase very likely would be delivered to us the next day.

Early the next morning, we received a call from Baggage Claim that they had our suitcase and would deliver it in the morning. Blossom and I were both taking courses at Skidmore College in Saratoga and would not be home, so I told them I would leave the side door of the garage open. The driver could leave the suitcase in the garage.

When we returned home in the afternoon, there was no suitcase in the garage. We also noticed that the garbage collector had taken our garbage, although we had forgotten this was the day for the pick up. I immediately called Baggage Claim in Albany and was informed that the driver had left the suitcase as instructed. Then, suspecting the suitcase may have been taken accidentally by the garbage collector, I called the garbage company. They said there was no chance of recovery if it had been taken with the garbage since it would be compacted. I asked them to question the pick-up person, but they obtained no information. I just couldn't believe anyone could mistake a brand-new suitcase for garbage.

The next step was to contact my insurance company. They told me to submit an inventory of the contents, which were quite valuable, and they would reimburse us. Having told them the story, I was surprised and inquired why didn't they conduct an investigation to try to find out what happened.

The reply was that an investigation would cost more than just reimbursing us. We were reimbursed, except for the deductible, but we did lose some of our best, favorite clothes.

With great anticipation in January 1986, we flew to San Francisco on the first leg of our trip to Australia and New Zealand. We were met by our friends Shirley and Edgar Miller and were guests in their home in Redwood City. We had a most enjoyable time visiting and being shown the Bay Area, including Stanford University.

We embarked from the San Francisco Airport on an AARP-chartered plane on which were members of our particular tour group. Since AARP sponsored several groups at the same time, they could fill the plane with their travelers. It was a long trip to Sydney, Australia, with only a fueling stop in Hawaii. The wisdom of our stopover in California was proven by the extreme exhaustion of those who had started the trip on the East Coast.

On about our third day in Sydney, Blossom received a phone call from California that her sister Razie (Razelle) had died. After our Thanksgiving visit, we had learned that she had cancer of the colon with metastases to the lung. She was not expected to recover, but at the time we left in January, she was not considered terminal.

We were faced with a dilemma. We were anxious to attend the funeral, but it would have been exhausting and would completely disrupt our trip. Blossom called back and talked to members of the family about returning for the funeral. They were very understanding and encouraged us to stay in Australia and continue our trip. We talked it over between us and decided to stay. In making the decision, it helped that we had spent a good deal of time with Razie when she was in the hospital during our Thanksgiving visit.

It was the first loss of a brother or sister for either of us, and it was a difficult time for Blossom. The first call came when we were having breakfast with our group and was announced as an emergency call for Blossom Friedman. Although we had only known our traveling companions for a few days, when word spread about the death, we suddenly became a family. The group arranged a memorial service and donated to a fund that would be contributed to the American Cancer Society. This outpouring of affection and sympathy was most supportive, and Blossom appreciated it and coped very well.

On one of our free days, we and another couple went to a municipal golf course, rented clubs, and enjoyed playing a round of golf. Golf courses abound in Australia, as noted when flying over the countryside.

Our basic program for three weeks included Sydney, Melbourne, and Kangaroo Island. We had been warned that Kangaroo Island would be primitive, and it was. The men and women were separated and slept in different compounds. Six of us slept in a small room with three bunk beds. I slept very well because when I take out my hearing aids at night, sounds don't bother me. However, in the morning, some of the men complained about loud snoring that disturbed their sleep, and they arranged to go to another bunk.

On the third week of our trip while on Kangaroo Island, Blossom fractured her ankle. This handicapped her for the rest of the trip, but she was stoical by nature and kept going.

After our basic three-week program was completed, our group broke up, with many returning home. I asked some of our colleagues why they had not chosen to stay and continue on some elective programs since it was such a long trip to get to Australia. To my surprise, I was told that three weeks was as long as they could stay away without paying bills and attending to their homes and personal matters. This made me feel proud of the program I had devised allowing us to stay away for the entire winter.

One of the courses of study in Australia dealt with the Australian entertainment industry, especially the movies. Their attempt at making movies was a fledgling enterprise with a distinct sense of inferiority to the great American movie industry. Much has changed since 1986, however, as demonstrated by the Oscars being awarded recently to the Australians, Russell Crowe and Nicole Kidman, for best actor and actress.

We were now on our own for the remainder of our stay, although our tours were mapped out for us. We flew from Sydney to Auckland, New Zealand, to start our tour of this country. It has more greenery than Australia and supports the major sheep-raising industry. It is a fascinating country to visit with hot springs, mountains, fjords, and the interesting city of Christchurch, which appears like a typical city in England.

The most exciting day in New Zealand occurred when we flew from Queenstown to Milford Sound. The world-famous attractions at Milford Sound are the fjords. We chose to fly on a small plane rather than take a long bus trip from Queenstown and return the same way. Obviously, the pilot had a great deal of experience and confidence because he thrilled us by flying between the glaciers on the way. It seemed like the tips of the wings almost touched the glaciers. At Milford Sound, we boarded a tour boat for a cruise showing us the fjords. We greatly enjoyed the day and the return flight.

After completing our tour of New Zealand, we were in the Auckland Airport waiting for our flight back to Australia. Something was fouled up with the seating on the plane, and people were called up one by one to be assigned a seat and board the plane. Everybody was boarded, but three couples, including us, remained in the waiting room. We were concerned, since it seemed we were going to be bumped. Then, we were reassured by an official that we were going to be seated in the first-class section since the coach section was full. It was a very welcome break because Blossom's ankle was hurting, and there, she was able to elevate her foot while we enjoyed the drinks, food, and service.

Our tour then took us to the outback, the sparsely inhabited area of Australia where the city of Alice Springs is located. In this area is the famous Ayers Rock, which is best remembered by me as the site of the thickest collection of flies I ever experienced. To service this isolated mountain was a beautiful, modern Sheraton Hotel, for which we were pleased and thankful.

Then we flew to Cairns, a city that provides access to the Great Barrier Reef and sugar plantations. It was hot and humid there. This was the last place we visited before preparing for our departure to return to the United States after an extremely worthwhile and enjoyable trip.

Chapter 36

On our return flight, we had arranged a stopover of three days in Honolulu, Hawaii. We had not spent time in this city on our previous visit. In this way, we broke up the long flight to Los Angeles, had a chance to rest after our strenuous tours, and then went sightseeing. Most impressive was the Pearl Harbor Memorial where the battleship *Arizona* lies on the bottom.

We also visited the Bishop Museum, named after the princess and wife of Charles Reed Bishop, who was a native of Glens Falls. They were married in 1850, and he became the power behind the throne and very prominent in business and banking in Hawaii.

From Hawaii, we flew to Southern California, where we remained until the beginning of April.

We always anticipated returning to Glens Falls and now our home in Queensbury each spring, where we would be back with our friends and family and could enjoy the natural beauty of this region.

The years 1985 and 1986 were important in the development of my intent to pioneer the improvement of the understanding of the aging process for the people of this area. One of my pleasures and best learning experiences when attending scientific meetings relating to gerontology was to watch the wonderful moving pictures that were presented on related subjects. Since most of these movies could be understood and appreciated by the lay public, I felt that a program presenting them at a public forum like the ones held at Crandall Library would be a valuable and acceptable way to disseminate needed information.

In the early summer of 1985, I contacted Christine McDonald, the very enlightened director of Crandall Library, and presented my proposal for a film series on aging. She agreed that this would be a worthwhile program to present and assigned Carol Whitcher, the outreach coordinator of the library who was trying to develop more programs for the aging, to work with me in the planning. *The Post-Star* was cooperative in providing publicity, and the following is the published interview I gave to the paper before the first program:

STEREOTYPES ON AGING UNTRUE: GERONTOLOGIST

BY SHEILA MAGEE NASON
Staff Writer

Dr. Orel Friedman says that only about 25 percent of the aging will ever end up in nursing homes.

This means, he emphasizes, that 75 percent will not. Friedman says it is commonly believed that the aging are forgetful, confused, fragile and in ill health, blind and deaf, asexual with no interest in sexuality and dependent. These stereotypes are all untrue for the majority of the aging, he said.

He prefers the term aging to senior citizen, elderly or mature.

"Life is a continuing process. If you are going to live, you're going to become one of the aging", he says.

Friedman, who has specialized in gerontology since he retired five years ago from his ear, nose and throat practice, will be presenting a special film series on the aging at Crandall Library. Each film will be followed by a brief lecture and a discussion period.

The first presentation, from 7 to 8:30 p.m. Wednesday, will be on "Intergenerational Programs." The film documentary will depict an intergenerational chorus comprised of members from 9 to 90 who came together through the efforts of an elementary school music teacher. Friedman says the discussion will concentrate on the importance of bringing the aging together with those of other generations in a variety of activities.

The second program, "Sexuality in the Later Years," will be from 7 to 8:30 p.m. Sept. 11. Friedman said 60 percent of men between 60 and 70 are capable of having sexual relations and that 40 percent of those between 70 and 80 are capable. He said society tends to express its opinion of the continued desire of the aging for loving relationships by telling jokes about "dirty old men."

A program from noon to 1:30 p.m. Wednesday, Sept.18, will be "Physical Fitness in the Later Years." Friedman said aging persons participate in a variety of physical activities, including yoga, dancing, running, swimming and tennis.

The program from 7 to 8:30 p.m., Monday Sept. 23, will cover "Pre-Retirement Planning and Retirement."

The final program in the series, Alzheimer's Disease," will be from noon to 1:30 p.m. Monday, Sept. 30.

The film series was developed jointly by Friedman and Carol Whitcher, outreach coordinator at the library. It is being financed through partial funding from the Southern Adirondack Library System.

Mrs. Whitcher, who visits Stichman Towers, the Cronin High Rise and area nursing homes for Crandall Library, is trying to develop more programs for the aging. Friedman was born in Glens Falls and is a graduate of the Glens Falls High School. He received his MD degree from Albany Medical College and conducted an ear, nose and throat practice here for 30 years. Five years ago, a serious eye problem caused him to give up his practice.

He says he discovered he was retired and that he was not prepared for it. He went to Crandall Library and began reading up on the subject, developing such a strong interest that he decided to start a second career in gerontology. He worked in group counseling with a psychologist, attended national meetings, served a 10 week internship in aging services at a mental health clinic in Florida and took a course at the State University of New York on working with the elderly.

Friedman practiced in the field for part of one year. He says he then realized he had to make a choice. If he wanted to stay in full-time practice, he would have to stay in Glens Falls every winter. He and his wife, Blossom, preferred to travel.

In recent winters they have been in Florida, Spain and Israel, and they will be spending this winter on an Elderhostel program in Australia.

But when he is in Glens Falls, Friedman continues to lecture on the subject of aging, trying to create a more optimistic attitude about the subject.

He said the aging are the fastest growing group in the United States. More than 5000 Americans celebrate their 65th birthday every day, and more than 30 million have passed this milestone.

He said the social, health and economic problems resulting in this tremendous increase in the elderly population make it important for every age group to be informed on the subject. The programs he will be presenting are designed to appeal to the young and the middle-aged, as well as the aging, he said.

All programs in the series are free and open to the public. Handicapped parking and entrance are located on the Maple Street side of the building."

The film program was very successful with a large, enthusiastic attendance and interesting discussions. The final program on Alzheimer's disease was most exciting for me because many of the people attending had been or were, at that time, caregivers for family members with Alzheimer's disease. Listening to their comments was a great learning experience for me and all in attendance.

The following September, we repeated the program with the presentation of a new set of films. Janice Kernan, the new outreach coordinator, assisted in the arrangements. I was interviewed again, this time by Joan Martinelli, staff writer for *The Post-Star*. The following article appeared on September 27, 1986:

AGE-OLD PROBLEM

FILM-LECTURE SERIES SEEKS TO DISPEL MYTHS OF AGING

People should look forward to aging with anticipation, not trepidation, according to Dr. Orel Friedman.

Friedman will be coordinating the film-lecture series, "Aging: A Celebration of Life," five consecutive Monday evenings starting tonight at Crandall Library.

"I'm very anxious to have young and middle-aged people attend the programs," he said. "There isn't enough contact between the generations. Consequently younger people just don't know what's ahead for them. Middle-aged people have these myths and stereotypes impressed in their minds that the aging are all ending up in rocking chairs or wheelchairs, and they face aging with trepidation."

The more contact generated between different age groups, the better for everyone, Friedman believes. By the year 2025 every sixth American will be over 65.

"Today a person 65 may have a quarter of his life ahead of him," he said. *"What we want to emphasize is that the vast majority of the aging are physically active, mentally alert, caring, independent, useful human beings."*

The aged still have tremendous contributions to make, Friedman said. *"A person 65 is equivalent to someone much younger a generation or two ago. We're in much better shape now, even up to the age of 80."* After that, the condition may begin to deteriorate, he said.

The time will come when a spouse or the family has to cope with illness or death. *"Families often haven't had much experience with death and dying,"* Friedman said.

"In the distant past, people had to take care of their own. Birth and death were just part of life. Now both generally happen in a hospital, and we are protected from this part of life, and I think that's a mistake."

The overall series will put aging into perspective as a time to celebrate life. The programs will focus on retirement, intergenerational relationships, family relationships, crime protection and quality of life.

"Many people are forced into retirement," he said, *"and even more face it unprepared. The day you first go to work, you should really start planning,"* Friedman said, *"but certainly by the time you reach your winter years.*

"If 65 is an age people retire, and that's very arbitrary, they should start thinking about retirement planning at age 50."

The three main areas to plan for are finances, health care and leisure time, he said.

"When you start planning years and years ahead, you're much better off," said Friedman. "If you retire and then say, 'Well, now I am gonna start playing golf and I'm gonna start square dancing, fishing, or start anything-writing, crocheting or making quilts, whatever the activity,' if you wait too long it's more difficult to get started. It's much easier to get discouraged."

"Our purpose is to show that retirement can result in rejuvenation," Friedman said. Some people use the time to embark on a second career, do volunteer work, travel or participate in educational programs.

"It is important to do things that are meaningful," he said, "not to do things for 'busy work' to be occupied. In the long run, 'busy work' won't give you the satisfaction to make life worth enjoying."

"Successful pre-retirement planning is a couple activity," Friedman said. "People go through married life raising a family, spouses go off to occupations making social contacts through the office. They really have been living together but not doing a lot of things together. That's all right as long as they both are so busy that they don't have time to think about what they are not doing."

But all of a sudden people find themselves with all this time together. "There is a sort of a honeymoon period," Friedman said. A husband probably has a million chores around the house to catch up on. So for six months, maybe nine, he's busy painting and fixing up and doing all these things he has neglected. But then if he has nothing else, and has no work to go to, eventually he may be sitting around the house with nothing to do."

If the wife was a homemaker, Friedman pointed out, her daily routine probably hasn't changed, including her social contacts. "She may still be busy, and the guy doesn't know what to do with himself. It can become a source of great friction," he said.

"It's amazing how people go through life raising their family, and they've got their jobs, and they are worrying about money

and this and that, but they never talk to each other about themselves, about how they feel about things and what they hope to do."

Friedman is here to tell everyone that retirement can be a wonderful time, but it takes some careful planning.

"That's how I feel about it," he said, "and that's what I am trying to impart-just how to accomplish that."

The series, "Aging: A Celebration of Life," will be presented from 7 to 8:30 to-night and for the following four consecutive Mondays in the library auditorium."

The films for the program are: "Active Retirement," "Intergenerational Relationships," "Family Relationships," "Crime Protection" and "The Good Long Life."

The film series was well received again, and plans were made to present another series the following year. When we started our planning, we found that the nights we wanted would not be available, and we decided to skip one year and return the next one. However, this resulted in a loss of momentum and interest, and eventually, we decided not to continue.

I was very happy with the reception the film series received, and I enjoyed the challenge of conceiving and bringing it to fruition. For me, it represented a significant advance in my desire to bring accurate, positive information about aging to the residents of this area. I had come a long way from my retirement disaster six years previously.

Chapter 37

In 1986, I began writing a booklet describing the methods used to take care of our home and personal and financial affairs while we were abroad for three or more months during the winter. I continued to work on the booklet in Florida where we spent the 1986-87 winter.

We chose to go to the West Coast to Punta Gorda, a city in South Florida. We rented an apartment in a complex where my cousin Frank LeVine lived all year with a dog for a companion. Frank was a widower and did not socialize at all. He spent his time fishing, reading a great deal, and watching television.

We had a very enjoyable time there and played considerable golf. Frank joined us when we went out to dinner and when we socialized with some of the people we met. We enjoyed his company, and he let us know that the time spent with us was the best he had experienced in a long time.

Frank owned a motor boat and a large recreational vehicle and decided to sell both of them. He found a customer interested in the boat in Fort Myers, so he drove the boat there by going out to the Gulf of Mexico. He made the sale and arranged for the boat to be picked up by the customer later that day in Punta Gorda. The two men who bought the boat would ride back with him and meet their wives in Punta Gorda, where they would come by car. However, on his return, there was a storm, and it was unsafe to try to bring the boat from the gulf through the inlet and then home. They were forced to leave the boat at a marina on the coast and make other arrangements for its delivery.

While we had no knowledge of the deal or what had happened, Blossom and I noticed two women driving around and then parking as if they were looking for someone in Frank's area. We asked if we could help them, and they told us they were waiting for Frank and their husbands, who were coming by boat, and should have been there by this time. Eventually, they made contact and went to pick up the men.

Early the next morning, Frank called us and asked if we would help him retrieve the boat, which he still could not drive through the inlet. We agreed, and the three of us started out with a large boat trailer he had obtained attached to the back of his large recreational vehicle. When we reached the marina, we found that the storm had knocked out the electrical power, and the winch which was used to pull the boat out and help place it on the trailer was not working. It was not possible to pull the boat out manually there, but we were informed that the boat could be driven to a beach a few miles away where we could pull it out of the water.

Frank would drive the boat, and he asked us to drive this monster vehicle with a trailer to the other beach. Neither of us had ever driven such a vehicle, and the attached trailer compounded the problem. We looked at each other, and Blossom said she would try to drive it after being given a crash course on how to do it. We were given directions to our destination, and off we went. Blossom was handling the vehicle well, but then we missed a turn in the town and had to turn around. This presented a real problem, so we drove around until we found a fairly large parking lot near a school that was empty because it was a weekend. I went outside, and Blossom blindly turned the vehicle and trailer around, following my directions and gesticulations without damaging the vehicle from a hit by the trailer. This was quite an experience, and finally, we reached our destination where Frank had been waiting for a long time, wondering where we were.

He backed the trailer into the water, and the three of us had to wade in the water to pull the boat on the trailer. It was hard work, but we finally got the boat on the trailer, which was too large for the boat and hard to stabilize on it when it was tied down.

Finally, with a sigh of relief, we headed for home, with the trailer swinging rather wildly, and, after a harrowing trip, reached our dock. Again, we had to work hard to get the boat in the water. With the job finished, we headed to our apartment exhausted and hungry but laughing about our unforgettable experience.

We enjoyed our stay in Punta Gorda, and with the arrival of spring, we said goodbye to Frank and headed back to our home in Queensbury.

I completed the manuscript for my booklet to which I gave the name *Worry Free Vacations Abroad*. I could not find anyone interested in publishing it, since it was only fourteen pages long. Eventually, I found a young man starting a business called Secretarial Overflow Service (SOS) who agreed to publish and distribute the booklet. I wanted an attractive cover, and we hired an artist to design it. However, he procrastinated and was holding up the publication, so I fired him and asked Blossom to help me out using her artistic talent. She prepared an attractive black-and-white cover that was very suitable. We published two hundred copies and faced the problem of selling them.

I went to all the bookstores in the area, but no one was interested except for one chain bookstore in the Aviation Mall. They gave me the encouraging news that they would put ten copies of any publication by a local author on their bookshelves. This was a start.

At that time, I belonged to the American Association of Senior Physicians (AASP), an affiliate of the American Medical Association. I sent them a copy of the booklet and a covering letter, hoping they would mention it in their newsletter. They were impressed, and the following article appeared in the *AASP Newsletter*, April/May 1988, volume 13, number 2, page 5:

PHYSICIAN PROFILE

OREL FRIEDMAN, M.D.

We recently received an interesting letter from an AASP member living in Glens Falls, New York. Orel Friedman, M.D., is active in retirement, having retired in 1980 because of an eye problem, following a span of some 30 years as an Otolaryngologist.

Dr. Friedman states he was one who was not prepared for retirement. As a result of his eye problems, he realized he was retired whether he liked it or not. He did not have the opportunity to prepare his practice for sale, even though colleagues assisted him by seeing patients that had to have care during his illness. Within thirty days of his illness, Dr. Friedman realized he did not have a practice left, so he merely "closed the door of his office."

Not one to simply accept the lot that had befallen him and with subsequent improvement in his vision, Dr. Friedman began to "study retirement," reading a collection of books on the subject at his local library. He became interested in the subject, wishing to know as much as he could about aging and gerontology. He began attending seminars and courses on retirement and gerontology, even attending one of AASP's "Achieving A Successful Medical Retirement" course in 1981 in Sarasota, Florida. He then worked for a year in group counseling with a psychiatrist and spent a ten week internship in a community health center with an adult counseling service in Florida. Upon his return to Glens Falls, he began practicing gerontological counseling but decided he and his wife did not want to stay in Glens Falls through the winter seasons so he gave up that career.

Since then he has been free-lancing as a speaker on the subject, and for a time, presented a film series on aging at his local library.

Dr. Friedman is not one to permit grass to grow under his feet. He believes that retirement can and should result in rejuvenation, using one's retirement time to embark on a second career, do volunteer work, participate in educational programs or travel. During recent winters, he and his wife have been to Florida, Spain, Israel and in an Elderhostel program in Australia.

During his travels abroad, Dr. Friedman became aware of the need for information directed toward retirees to facilitate the handling of financial and personal affairs while being abroad for several months. So he did something about it-he authored a pamphlet "Worry Free Vacations Abroad" which outlines his proposals for problems relating to mail, banking, finances, taxes, securities and one's home while spending long vacations abroad. This pamphlet is available to anyone who *might find it helpful by writing: Secretarial Overflow Service, P.O. Box 600, Glens Falls, NY 12801 and enclosing a check for $3.50 per copy, payable to "Worry Free Vacations Abroad."*

Dr. Friedman is also in the process of writing a short story on "Death and Dying." In addition, he was recently appointed to serve on a Committee on Geriatric Otolaryngology for the American Academy of Otolaryngology-Head and Neck Surgery, Inc.

His "retirement" is an example of doing things that are meaningful, not merely doing things for "busy work" but rather those things that gives one satisfaction and makes life worth living. That is what retirement at its best is all about."

This article had very favorable results, and we received orders from physicians in all parts of this country. We sold out the first printing of two hundred copies and printed two hundred more. The bookstore sold the ten copies they had, but they told me sales were slow because interested people would read the entire small booklet and then return it to the shelf.

Shortly after the AASP article was published, I received a letter from Dr. Maxwell Ibsen of San Jose, California, who had served with me in the 93rd General Hospital in England during World War II, where he was in charge of the clinical laboratory. We met at Fort Meade, Maryland, shortly before going overseas, and I found out he had known Blossom in Philadelphia. He visited Blossom in Lebanon, Pennsylvania, with me on my only trip there before going overseas. I lost touch with him after the war, during which time he became a doctor of medicine. As a result of this contact, we enjoyed visiting him and his wife in San Jose on two occasions.

The booklet sales were doing nicely when the owner of Secretarial Overflow Service decided to go out of business. I didn't want to bother with the mail-order business, and sales faded out.

Just as my accomplishments as a public speaker and in presenting the film series were steps in the ladder of my success as an active retiree, so was the publication of *Worry Free Vacations Abroad.*

Chapter 38

I was already pursuing a new interest, the subject of death and dying, when my booklet, *Worry Free Vacations Abroad*, was published. For a considerable time, I had observed that end-of-life care in this country was a neglected branch of medicine and, in many cases, was abysmal.

Although in my specialized practice I did not care for many terminal patients, I was part of the system brought up on the use of all our modern technology to prolong life even if it only served to prolong the patient's suffering. The wishes of the dying person and their families were mostly ignored as long as there was another procedure that could be done to futilely extend life. The end-of-life care my mother received in 1975 was given by a compassionate physician using the standards of the time, but he prolonged her dying with an unnecessary terminal hospitalization. After my retirement and feeling released from the restraints of conforming and fearing lawsuits, I became more objective and viewed death and dying from more than one viewpoint.

I was greatly incensed by the end-of-life care given my 103-year-old aunt, my mother's sister, who had been a resident of a nursing home for several years. She was bedridden, blind, suffered from heart failure, and a gastrointestinal problem with alternating constipation and diarrhea. She begged her doctors to let her die, but instead, they would hospitalize her every time she had an acute flare-up of the underlying disease. It was a perfect example of technology triumphing over common sense and compassion for the incurable, unhappy 103-year-old woman. Since she was on Medicare and also Medicaid because all her money had been used up long before, her unnecessary, prolonged care was costing these services a great deal of money. Eventually, even technology could no longer prolong her life and suffering, and she died.

I had a great desire to publicize her story to demonstrate the sad state of end-of-life care in our country, which has the finest scientific and technological health-care system in the world. My approach was to write a fictionalized short story based on the terminal phase of my 103-year-old aunt's life. At that time, she did not have a living will, but in those early days, it would have probably been ignored even as they are sometimes today. In real life, there was no way for her to end her misery, but in the short story, which was given the title "Flight 30," a unique means of ending the misery of terminal patients was devised.

The title "Flight 30" was descriptive of a special one-way airplane flight for terminal or incurable patients from which there was no return. Even the flight personnel, while still able to function for this flight, had illnesses for which there was no hope. The airplane was a commercial plane that no longer met all the standards but was suitable for a short one-way flight. The number 30 is a newspaper term that is used at the finish of a submitted story and indicates the "end of the story." And that is what the one-way flight was meant to indicate. It was not necessary to elaborate further regarding what happened to the flight.

"Flight 30" was copyrighted in 1988 and was then submitted to a magazine for publication. It was rejected and then submitted to another. This process was repeated over and over for the next two years. It was very disappointing and frustrating, but not unusual for an unknown author submitting a short story highly critical of the medical establishment. I followed every lead and approached anyone of influence I knew for help in getting my story published but without success.

I even submitted the story to Ann Landers, hoping she would find it worthwhile and help me find a publisher but to no avail. A prominent politician and educator expressed ideas similar to mine on a radio program, and I sent him "Flight 30," asking for help in getting it published. He graciously wrote me that my short story deserved publication, but he could not help me. He even sent me a short story of his own on end-of-life care that had not been published.

One "little magazine" wrote me a very encouraging letter and made some suggestions how the story could be improved, but they were ceasing publication and could not use it. I did incorporate their suggestions in future manuscripts that were submitted. All I had to show for all my effort was a great collection of rejection slips.

I now rationalize that my failure to get published was because my story was ahead of its time. Before 1990, when Dr. Kevorkian's first assisted suicide case was publicized, there was little interest in the insensitive approach to the prolonged and unnecessary suffering of the dying. The publicity resulting from his efforts to help terminal and incurable human beings obtain the relief that was being denied them eventually acted as a "wake-up call" to the medical profession, hospitals, the clergy, lawyers, and politicians that end-of-life care needed radical improvement. How could a society like ours call itself enlightened when it required a terminally ill, suffering person to leave the security and comfort of home and family and travel a long distance to another state where a perfect stranger would assist him or her in dying in a place like the back of a van? Dr. Kevorkian was influential in forcing the establishment to consider ways to improve end-of-life care.

Although my short story was never published, my interest in end-of-life care was very greatly aroused, and I began familiarizing myself with the organizations and literature promoting a caring, enlightened approach to this problem. I made a study of physician-assisted suicide and prepared a lecture on this subject that I presented to interested organizations, just as I had previously done in relation to aging. Both physician-assisted suicide (or the preferable term, physician-assisted death) and truly compassionate end-of-life care are causes that are worth fighting for and have been a consuming interest of mine to this very day.

It was time for Blossom and me to make plans regarding our next winter vacation, although we knew we wanted to spend it in Israel. In the summer of 1987, after our son Victor had obtained his doctor of education from Harvard University, he and Nurit planned to return to Israel with their three children to make their permanent home there. Many native Israeli women wanted to marry Americans and live in this country, but Nurit gave up a very responsible, well-paying job to return to the country she loved. Victor was totally in agreement with her, even though he could have had many opportunities in his field in America.

At the same time, our daughter Beverly Seligson and her husband, Joel, also decided to go to Israel to live there with their four children. They had met in Israel, married and then lived in Finland for about two years while he continued his education there. He is a brilliant scientist, and the University of Rochester offered him the financial support he needed to pursue a Ph.D. in physics, specializing in optics. After earning his degree, he worked for the Kodak Company for a few years. Beverly was busy during their years in Rochester, New York, giving birth to four daughters, raising them and working as a nurse. Since she loved working with food, she gave up nursing and established her own catering business. However, the Seligsons dreamed of living in Israel where they had met.

They decided to make *aliyah*, which means "going up" in Hebrew and means moving to Israel to live. They and Victor's family had reached an age when it was now or never. It helped that both families were going at the same time. We gave them a big farewell party before they left, and I recall saying, "I support your move because this is something you have thought about doing for a long time. If you don't go now, you will wonder for the rest of your lives whether you made a mistake and missed out on a worthwhile and important life experience."

We wanted to spend our next winter in Israel near our families. Knowing that Hadassah sponsored a two-month volunteer program called Winter in Netanya (WIN), similar to the B'nai B'rith ARI program we had participated in previously, we signed up for the WIN program. After we completed our volunteer program, we planned to rent an apartment and spend two more months in Netanya.

We left for Israel in December 1988 and enjoyed our WIN experience. This time, we stayed at the lovely Blue Bay Hotel in the northern section of Netanya. I again worked as a volunteer in the old-age and nursing home, where they were pleased to have me return. It was another positive experience for us, and we had the pleasure of seeing our children and grandchildren as often as possible. We did rent an apartment for the two months as planned and enjoyed being on our own, shopping for food, sightseeing, and visiting with family and the friends we had made in Israel.

Victor had a longtime close friendship with Thomas L. Friedman, a Pulitzer Prize-winning foreign correspondent for *The New York Times*, stationed at that time in Jerusalem. Their friendship began when they were students at Brandeis University. Tom had told us to contact him if we came to Jerusalem, and on one of our visits there, we did. He and his lovely wife, Ann, invited us to go to dinner with them, and on a pleasant, sunny day, Tom drove us to a favorite restaurant of his in Jericho, in the West Bank. It was a most enjoyable experience spending the day with them.

Soon, it was spring and time to return home. As much as we enjoyed being in Israel and near our family, we never seriously thought of going there to live. We met many aging couples who were living in Israel because they wanted to be near their children. Although we had played golf many times at Israel's only golf facility, an excellent course in Caesarea, not far from Netanya and Zichron Yaakov, where Victor and Nurit lived, being a member there did not have the same appeal as the Glens Falls Country Club. I had difficulty learning Hebrew, especially because of my hearing problem, and would have difficulty communicating. We could visit our children in Israel from time to time, and they would be coming to visit us. Also, we had our daughter Barbara and her family living in New York City. We were happy and comfortable with our lifestyle in the United States and had no desire to change.

On my return home from my winter vacation, I returned to serving on the Utilization Review Committee of three local nursing homes. We met for about an hour once a month to carry out some state mandates regarding the classification of level of care required for the residents in the facility. Also, we discussed the quality of care and how to maintain and improve it. My knowledge of gerontology was very useful, and it was also a learning experience and something I enjoyed. I became acquainted with nurses and administrators, and I enjoyed being with them and other physicians who served on these boards. I received a small stipend for this work, and they welcomed me back each year after I returned from my winter vacation. To save money, the state eliminated positions like mine several years ago.

I felt very good about the quality of nursing-home care provided by these facilities and their personnel for the people of our area.

It seems that coming home meant starting to think about and planning for our next winter's adventure.

Chapter 39

We had been to Mexico twice before as tourists, but our very good friends Dr. Jacques and Hilda Grunblatt from North Creek, New York, aroused our interest in spending a winter there.

Jacques was a unique individual with a most interesting background. He was born in Poland and attended medical school in France. When the Spanish civil war broke out, he joined the International Brigades of the Republican army fighting against the dictator Franco. With the defeat of his army, he was interned in France. He eventually escaped and came to Mexico, where he practiced medicine until 1946 when he came to the United States. He met Hilda in Brooklyn, New York, and after they were married, they moved to North Creek.

He practiced there for many years until he suffered a severe heart attack which forced him to retire. Because Mexico took him in when no one else would, he had a special attachment to that country. After his retirement, he and Hilda spent several long winters in Manzanillo, a quiet resort city on the west coast of Mexico, the so-called Mexican Riviera. The Grunblatts extolled the wonderful climate, the beaches, and low cost of living there. They told us there were golf courses in the area.

Manzanillo sounded like a delightful place to spend the winter. Our friends advised us to make a reservation for a few days in a hotel near where they stayed and use this as a base to look for an apartment for the three months we planned to stay. The golf courses were situated in another part of the city, and they suggested that it would be more convenient for us to live in that area.

We followed their advice and made plans to visit our family in California before going to Mexico. We arrived in Manzanillo in the early evening, checked into our hotel, and walked outside toward a restaurant that had been recommended to us. In doing so, we passed and recognized the name of the cottage colony where the Grunblatts stayed. Since it was getting late, we decided to drop in on them, say hello briefly, make plans for the next day, and leave.

When I rang the doorbell, the Grunblatts' son Jesse opened the door and greeted me very warmly. We entered the house and saw the entire family there, but not Jacques. They told us that he had just died and had been buried that day in Manzanillo in accordance with his request, since he had such affection for Mexico. What had been planned as a friendly visit turned out to be a condolence call, and we felt privileged that fate had allowed us to bring whatever comfort we could to this bereaved family of friends so far from home and any support group.

We met the next day, and they were making plans to leave. We said goodbye and then began exploring the city. We found an apartment colony which had one of the two golf courses in the city, and since one had to live in the complex to play the course, we rented a very nice apartment there.

One day, Blossom was lying on a couch around the swimming pool when a neighbor told her she was in a dangerous place because a coconut could fall and hit her. We started a conversation and asked him if he and his wife played bridge. They didn't, but they had come there from California with several couples, and one couple plays bridge. Later that day, the bridge players approached us, and we arranged a game.

We hit it off very well and also began golfing together. All the other couples left, but they stayed considerably longer, and we spent a good deal of time with one another. Also, the group had a large quantity of food left over, and our friends were left with it. We helped them finish it off. Because they had been coming to Manzanillo for years, they knew all about rentals. They informed us that a lovely studio apartment was available on the second floor of a private home where the rent was considerably cheaper than what we were paying. Also, we could still have golf privileges when staying there. We looked it over, rented, and moved.

The home was owned by a wealthy Mexican couple. In Mexico, homes are built that way in case one of the couple dies, and if the survivor has financial difficulties, he or she can move upstairs and get a good rental income from the main house.

Our newfound friends told us that they had a daughter in San Diego, California, who was an oncologist. Blossom's sister Adelle had died from cancer of the breast, and we had met her oncologist in San Diego because we spent considerable time with Adelle and her family before her death. I took one look at our friend's face, and I recognized Adelle's oncologist because of their resemblance. She was her mother.

She even knew about Adelle because Adelle and her husband had a high-class gift store in San Diego, and they had given a very attractive glass bowl to her doctor in appreciation for her caring attention. Naturally, she showed it to her mother. We had another bond in common.

Her daughter, the oncologist, was also a gourmet cook, and on a subsequent visit to San Diego, the daughter invited us to her home for dinner where we met her husband and her family. Her parents came in from their home in another city to be with us again.

After our newfound friends left for home, we enjoyed the company of other people we had met. The home we were in had the best possible water-purifying system, and we had the luxury of drinking water right out of the tap with impunity. We were careful where and what we ate out and used antiseptic drops in the water with which we rinsed our vegetables and fruits at home. Fortunately, neither of us had a bad moment.

The weather during our three months stay was gorgeous with temperature in the 70s and no humidity. On one day only was there a small amount of rain. Our new apartment was only one block away from an excellent beach, and I started going to the beach and swimming, something I thought I had given up forever. We also did some traveling and sightseeing during our stay in Mexico. We returned home in the spring after an idyllic winter vacation not knowing that it would be our last one together.

Chapter 40

Our return plane tickets required us to return to California before returning east, and we spent an enjoyable couple of weeks with family there.

On arriving back home, we were ready to get into our routine of visits to the dentist and doctors.

Blossom had a routine annual physical examination with laboratory studies, which showed she was anemic. Although she had not had any obvious bleeding from any source, her history of ulcers of the stomach in the past aroused suspicion. However, she had been symptom free since her subtotal gastrostomy many years previously. There were no findings on physical examination, so a gastroscopy (an examination of the stomach using a flexible electrically lighted tube) was performed. This revealed some shallow ulcers of the stomach but no obvious bleeding, and it was assumed that this was the probable cause of the anemia.

She was placed on a regimen of treatment for ulcers of the stomach and followed for several weeks, but the anemia was not improved. Although Blossom had been active during the summer playing golf and engaging in her usual activities, she began to complain of increasing fatigue and lack of energy.

We also had to make a decision about going to California in September to attend the wedding of our niece, Kathy Frank. Since the death of Kathy's mother, Blossom's sister Adelle, Blossom was like a surrogate mother to her. When we were in California in the spring of 1989, we had promised Kathy we would be there for her marriage, which was planned for September. Although Blossom was not feeling very well, she insisted on going to the wedding even though it would drain her energy and be very tiring. Kathy would have been very disappointed if we did not come, and since family ties and attending family functions were of great importance to both of us, we made the trip.

Another gastroscopy had been advised and was put on hold until after our return from California. We had a very enjoyable time at the wedding, and Kathy was overjoyed that we were there. Since this turned out to be Blossom's last trip to California and the opportunity to be with most of her family, the occasion was a blessing. We even talked about spending the next winter in Florida, where we would see many family members.

Toward the end of September, another gastroscopy was performed on Blossom. There was no evidence of significant change, and biopsies were taken in the area of the ulcers. The report showed cancer, and our lives would be changed forever.

By this time, she was having some difficulty eating, and I believe she had a definite premonition that the diagnosis would be cancer. Although her nature was to be optimistic, she knew that the females in her immediate family, her mother and her two sisters, had all died of cancer. Because of this history, for years she had seriously informed me, when discussing the future, that she would very likely predecease me. Especially during the years of my retirement, she made a conscious effort to prepare me to be able to survive without her. She would say jokingly but meaningfully, "I want you to know all these things so after I'm gone, you won't have to fall for the first woman who brings you a casserole."

I actually enjoyed doing most of the food and other shopping, and often, the supermarket would turn out to be the social center where I enjoyed meeting and talking to people. One of the advantages of retiring in my hometown was the many people I knew and enjoyed talking to. Blossom used to kiddingly complain, "I can't send you to the supermarket because you never come home."

One of the great benefits of my knowledge of gerontology was that over the years, I had gained much insight into the experience and the personality traits that would help or hinder the adjustment of a surviving spouse to being alone. Therefore, I was anxious to know everything about the kitchen and housekeeping as I could.

One thing she wanted to teach me was ironing, but I resisted. Later on, I was sorry.

When the diagnosis of cancer of the stomach was made, I knew the prognosis was poor, especially when it appeared that she had metastases to the retroperitoneal lymph nodes, an inaccessible area. Blossom was a very strong person and maintained her composure despite the gravity of the situation. The question was how to explain to her the approach to treatment that would offer her comfort and possible recovery. Although recovery appeared very unlikely, I could not be negative in my approach and support. To make it possible for her to continue eating, she underwent a very sophisticated operation to open her digestive track so she could eat. However, the cancer was not completely eliminated.

Her postoperative recovery was rapid, and on the day of her discharge from the hospital, we had a visit from friends from California. We went out to dinner, and to our amazement, Blossom enjoyed eating a hamburger sandwich without difficulty.

The next step was to treat the remaining cancer. Radiation therapy with minimal use of chemotherapy was recommended. However, the therapy was very discomforting, with no obvious improvement. One day, Blossom asked me point blank whether she should continue, and I honestly told her if she wanted to quit the therapy, I would support her decision without any reservations. She chose to discontinue all attempts at cure. Her general condition was deteriorating.

I was concerned about our relationship with our children and grandchildren in Israel, since it would have been difficult for everyone to come to America to see her. My suggestion was for us to go to Israel while it was still possible for her to make the trip frankly to say goodbye. Blossom was hesitant, however, because her physical appearance had changed so much. She thought it might be better if they remembered her at her best. We could not come to an agreement, and I suggested that we consult the leader at Caritas, the organization in the area assisting the seriously and terminally ill. Blossom had been a volunteer on the staff of Caritas, had great respect for this counselor, and agreed to seek her advice. The counselor supported my point of view, and we made plans for the trip. In early December 1989, we flew to Israel on El Al Airline with Blossom traveling in a wheelchair. We went business class, and the flights both ways were uneventful.

The visit turned out to be everything I had hoped for. As a family, we had always enjoyed being together telling stories and jokes and savoring good food. Blossom had a wonderful way with children, especially her grandchildren, and she and the grandchildren enjoyed every moment together. We laughed a lot and cried a little. Everyone sensed that this was the last time they would see Bubbe, and Bubbe knew this as well. Every moment together was precious.

On the evening of our departure for home, we all had dinner together and said our goodbyes. It was a time I will always remember as a highlight of our lives. It was a sad moment but very meaningful, containing all the love and pathos of a family coming together in the face of the impending death of the family's matriarch. That evening is forever etched in my memory.

Our trip home went well, and we arrived home a few days before the end of December. Our daughter Barbara and grandson Eitan came from New York City to spend the weekend with us. On Saturday evening, the four of us went to the country club for dinner. Blossom was weak, uncomplaining as usual, and still able to eat. We had a good time. Barbara and Eitan left the next day.

Blossom's condition deteriorated rapidly, and she died suddenly two days later.

Chapter 41

The death of a loved one is always sad. When a death occurs suddenly, it is tragic, and the deceased's suffering is usually minimal. It is very traumatic for friends and family because it is not anticipated and thus surprising.

When a death occurs after a long, lingering, often-painful illness, the opposite is the rule. The deceased has suffered for a long time, but the death has been anticipated. Family and friends have had an opportunity to say goodbye to the ill person and prepare psychologically for the death.

Blossom's death was neither sudden or the result of a long period of suffering. It occurred approximately three months after her operation for stomach cancer. If we had had a hospice program here at the time, she would undoubtedly have entered the program since she had stopped taking any therapy and her life expectancy was less than six months. After working with hospice in the terminal care of her sister Adelle in California, Blossom was so impressed she became a volunteer with Caritas, a local support group.

At the expense of appearing callous, I accepted her death with equanimity. Immediately, there were so many matters for me to attend to on my own that I did not have time to dwell on my widower state. From my knowledge of the terminal course of cancer of the stomach, her future could have been one of months of extreme suffering. Blossom preferred death to a long, lingering illness and had fortunately said goodbye to her loving family, whom she loved so much. We had had frank discussions about our relationship and the future. Perhaps our friends were not quite prepared for what happened because Blossom was not a complainer and did not conduct herself as a person whose demise was imminent. My severe sense of loss was tempered by the knowledge that her suffering was over and that, fortunately, she had been spared months of distress with no loss of dignity to her life. Knowing her, if she had a choice, it would be to "let go."

Her funeral was conducted in a sensitive, meaningful manner by Rabbi Richard J. Sobel of Temple Beth El in the temple. Rabbi Sobel had great affection and admiration for Blossom as a person and as a leader in all her undertakings. He was very supportive and helpful during this stressful time and has been and still is a very close friend. Family and friends gathered from all over the country and from Israel for the funeral. Blossom was the first member of our family to be buried in our plot in the Temple Beth El Cemetery, which my brother Moe and I had purchased together years before.

We observed the custom of shivah, the traditional seven-day period of mourning where the family stays at home and has an open house for daily religious services and to receive visitors. Everyone was saddened and seemed to be quite spiritless. I was not comfortable with this on the second day because the atmosphere was tense and morbid. I decided this should be changed, and as is my custom when I am trying to get a group to relax, I told a couple of jokes. It worked like magic, and the gathering became more animated and more like our usual get-togethers. Rhoda Forrest, Blossom's closest friend in Glens Falls, came from her winter home in California for the funeral and was very sad. She told me that the moment I told those jokes, her mood quickly changed for the better, and the process of accepting and starting to move on began.

Shivah is a wonderful custom because for the first week, the surviving immediate family has company and people to help them cope with the changed family structure. The family is not alone. The hard part begins when everyone usually leaves when shivah is over.

While mourning the loss of my beloved wife, when everyone left, I felt that I was as well prepared to live my new lifestyle as a widower as anyone could be. I was not depressed or fearful of what lay ahead. My positive mood resulted from my realistic nature, insight gained from my years in gerontology and counseling experience, and the knowledge of housekeeping and cooking that Blossom had instilled in me. A big plus was our housekeeper and friend, Joan Stegman, who had worked for us for years and whom I could depend on to come in every week for housekeeping and to do my laundry. During the shivah, my daughters also gave me practical cooking tips.

A few days after the shivah ended, I called up my golfing buddies and asked them to join me for lunch at the country club. When we were together, I could sense that they were somewhat ill at ease and not sure about what to say, so I broke the ice by telling a couple of jokes. Everyone felt more comfortable, and we had a good time.

We were joined by another friend who had lost his wife two years previously and was still mourning and feeling sorry for himself. He began to talk about her and cry, and I tried to cheer him up. His behavior did not upset me particularly nor spoil my attempt to get back to normal living.

I found comfort in attending temple services, as was my custom, and joining my friends there and have continued to make Temple Beth El an important part of my life to this day.

A few weeks after Blossom's death, the Super Bowl football game was scheduled, and I did not want to watch it alone. Fortunately, a Super Bowl party was scheduled at the country club, and I signed up to attend. Everybody there went out of their way to see that I had a good time, and I did. I was happy that I went.

Blossom and I had played bridge, but I found myself without anyone to play with. Taking a bridge course is a good way to meet people with whom you can continue playing after the lessons are over. We had taken a course several years previously from Marion Policastro, so I called her up, told her my problem, and asked about taking a course. She told me that she was no longer teaching but was in charge of a weekly duplicate bridge game at the Glens Falls Senior Center. Marion invited me to come there, and she would find me a partner. I went there that week and am still playing in that game.

It was winter, but I had no desire to go to Florida or elsewhere for a warmer climate. I was awakening early in the morning and needed to exercise, so I began walking in Aviation Mall with the early birds. Rabbi Sobel was often there, as were other acquaintances, so it was a combined exercise and social program.

I had my brother Moe and his wife, Janet, and their family in Schroon Lake for support. Dr. Leonard Busman and his wife, Mildred, in Bolton Landing, who had been our very close friends, generously included me in many of their social activities. I received many dinner invitations from friends, which I enjoyed and appreciated. I reciprocated by inviting them to lunch or dinner at the country club, which was always an excellent place to entertain guests. I had had a great deal of practice setting up meetings and dinners in organizational work, and entertaining came easily to me.

Time passed quickly, loneliness was never a problem, and I was doing very well cooking for myself and housekeeping. Of course, Joan Stegman was a great help with her weekly housekeeping and doing my laundry. Joan was Rhoda Forrest's regular housekeeper, and the Forrests were very good friends who were concerned about me. Rhoda used to question Joan about how I was getting along and then tell me, "You are the most independent person around," since there was little that they could do to help me in my adjustment.

Blossom and I were sexually active until her illness precluded sexual relations. As time passed and the pattern of my lifestyle was established, sexual frustration was a problem. I felt that my needs for companionship and socialization were being met very satisfactorily, and I was not interested in making a commitment for purely sexual reasons. At the time, women close to my age group did not attract me, and perhaps younger women might have appealed to me more. I just didn't travel in circles where there was an opportunity to meet younger women. I certainly was not aggressive in that respect.

It occurred to me that a prostitute would satisfy my needs, but at the same time, I knew that this was not a course for me because of personal fears and inhibitions. On the other hand, I fantasized that the type of social club and brothel as described by Polly Adler in her book *A House Is Not a Home* would be more to my taste. Of course, this was not realistic but made me wonder if perhaps there could be an acceptable place in our society to cater to the needs of men in the position that I found myself. After all, the play *The Best Little Whorehouse in Texas* found wide acclaim in America.

These thoughts may sound shocking, but until there is a need to be satisfied, the solution would not fit into the frame of reference of most of us. My problem was solved by the passage of time, and I have found my lifestyle as a single man very satisfying.

Chapter 42

Time passed quickly, and I decided to go to Florida in April and from there to Israel for the Passover holiday. I wanted to visit my sister Martha Schiffman and her husband, Leo. Blossom's brothers and their wives were also informed of my plans, and we arranged for all of us to get together in Palm Beach at the beautiful mansion of Ralph and Jacqueline Levitz. Sid and Bert Levitz came from California, Leon Levitz from Texas, and Sam and Lee Levitz from Arizona. Jackie and Ralph hosted a delightful party for the many family members who were in Florida. Ralph showed considerable disability as the result of the stroke he had suffered a few years previously.

Martha, Leo, and I drove to Palm Beach from their home in Deerfield Beach, about one hour away, where I was staying with them. Moe and Janet Friedman were in Florida, and they came.

It was the first time we were together since Blossom's funeral, and we talked about her and all the good times and family affairs of the past. There were tears and also a lot of laughs. The togetherness gave us all a lift and the realization that it was important to keep in touch with one another.

At the completion of my stay in Florida, I flew to Israel and spent Passover with my families there. My recollection is vague, but I believe Joel's parents, Lilli and Boris Seligson, from Finland were at the Seder with us. We were such good friends rather than just in-laws that it was always fun to be with them. It was very touching, because it was our first time together without Blossom.

While visiting with my children and grandchildren, the realization struck me that our last visit to Israel when Blossom was dying had been very important psychologically in preparing our family for her death. Only Victor and Beverly had come to America for the funeral, but the others had already said goodbye and, while saddened, were not traumatized. Gilead, aged three, had understood and said to me in an accepting manner, "Bubbe dead." Bubbe means grandmother in Yiddish and was the way the grandchildren referred to her. The way Gilead said this meant the world to me and never will be forgotten.

Although we were still grieving, we were going on with our lives and adjusting to the loss of our beloved Blossom—wife, mother, and grandmother. I was glad I made the trip and visit, and I returned home feeling good.

One of Blossom's great passions in life was her affiliation and very active participation in Hadassah, the women's Zionist organization and the largest Jewish women's organization in America. Because of her organizational, fund-raising, and leadership abilities, she had served on its National Board. I had been approached by friends in the Glens Falls chapter of Hadassah asking me for permission to have a tribute luncheon in Blossom's memory. This was also to be a fund-raising function for the benefit of the tissue-typing unit and the bone-marrow transplant department in the Hadassah Hospital in Jerusalem, Israel. I appreciated their desire to honor her memory, and the fund-raising was in keeping with Blossom's philosophy. She had often said, "If you are going to work hard to arrange an affair, why not raise money for a worthwhile cause so you'll have something to show for your effort." Of course, I approved and offered my support.

The tribute was held on Sunday, August 26, 1990, in the Queensbury Hotel in Glens Falls. There was an overflow attendance. The committee arranged an excellent program with two exceptional featured speakers.

One was Ruth W. Popkin, a former National President of Hadassah and at the time probably the most important woman in Jewish organizational life in the world. Barbara's mother-in-law, Sherley Plasse, is Ruth's very close friend from the days when Ruth lived in Great Neck, New York. Ruth is a widow, and we spent many good times with her, especially at holiday dinners in the Plasse home.

Victor asked his close friend Thomas L. Friedman, the distinguished author and Pulitzer Prize-winning columnist of *The*

New York Times, if he would speak at the tribute, and he readily agreed. Tom commands large fees for speaking but offered his services without charge as a favor to our family. As the chief diplomatic correspondent for *The New York Times* then covering the State Department, at the last minute, he found he could not come. It was the time when Saddam Hussein invaded Kuwait, and Tom called me the day before the affair and regretfully told me that since he was covering the Secretary of State, he could not leave Washington, D.C., at that crucial time. He was right, of course, but we were disappointed.

Ruth gave an inspiring talk and tribute to Blossom, as did other featured speakers, including our children, Barbara, Beverly, and Victor. Rhoda Forrest presented an excellent musical tribute. Janet Friedman presented the theme, reading "A Woman of Valor." The affair was an appropriate and moving tribute to Blossom.

The fund-raising was also very successful, and the money raised was added to the major contribution made by Leon Levitz, Blossom's brother, for the purpose of naming the tissue-typing unit and the bone-marrow transplant department in the Hadassah Hospital in Blossom's name.

The following summer, Leon, his daughter Linda, other family members and all our Orel Friedman family attended the moving ceremony for the formal dedication of the plaques in the Hadassah Hospital in Ein Karem, Jerusalem, Israel, naming the departments in Blossom's memory. It was another important occasion for our family to be together, even though we are divided between Israel and America.

Our daughter and son-in-law, Beverly and Joel Seligson, and their family also dedicated a wing of classrooms in their children's school in Blossom's memory. I attended the ceremony dedicating the plaque, and it was very moving and greatly appreciated.

After my visit to Florida in April 1990, I decided that I would spend several months in Florida the next winter in or near Deerfield Beach, where Martha and Leo Schiffman lived so we could spend time together. Also, Moe and Janet spent several winter months nearby.

When we spent the winter in Tampa, Florida, in 1981, Blossom and I looked at a villa in the Sarasota area that attracted us as a place where we might like to move to as a yearlong home. However, because I had not sold my practice and home-office property in Glens Falls and my finances were unsettled, to put it mildly, we did not dare commit ourselves to any purchase of property at that time or for the five years it took to finally sell.

After my second retirement, which was from counseling, at the end of 1981, we went to California for the winter and spent it with Blossom's sister Razie. We had a very good time and decided that instead of settling down in the same place every winter, it would be more enriching to spend several winter months in a different area or country each year. We had a wonderful time because almost every winter was a new and exciting experience.

After about ten years of going to different places, we were ready to start to thinking about looking for a winter home in Florida and doing less traveling. This was just before Blossom's final illness, which changed everything. However, my mental set was to winter in Florida, hopefully in a retirement residence where I could rent an apartment for the winter months.

When I was in Florida in April, my sister showed me a new, very attractive residence, the Forum, in Deerfield Beach, close to Century Village where she lived. This was just what I was looking for, but they would not commit themselves to renting on a part-time basis. They did put my name on their mailing list.

In the fall, when I contacted them, the Forum said they would not take anyone just for the winter. Then I was told by a friend in Glens Falls that a relative had lived in the Veranda Club in Boca Raton and had liked it. This was a senior residence not far from Deerfield Beach. Martha and Leo checked it out for me, and they liked it. They were willing to take me on a seasonal basis, and I signed up to go there. It was very desirable, and I liked living there. My neighbor across the hall was Viola Groat, a lovely person who introduced me to her son and his wife, Bill and Estelle Groat. Bill became my golfing partner in Florida for about ten years, along with his brother Jack, until Jack died a few years ago. We were all good friends and saw each other frequently. Viola Groat died a few years after I met her.

This first winter in Florida on my own proved to be very enjoyable. First, it took me away from the rigors of a Glens Falls winter, especially helpful because since my illness due to hyperthyroidism in 1979, I have had a low body temperature. I also developed Raynaud's disease which causes blanching and numbness of my fingers when they are exposed to cold. Warm weather is much more comfortable for me than cold weather.

I had plenty of relatives to be with in the area, like Martha and Leo, Moe and Janet, Ralph and Jackie Levitz, Esther Levitz, Philip and Margie Levitz. I found that by playing golf and bridge, I met new people to become friendly with. An independent-living retirement residence is an excellent place to meet people and make new friends, which I did at the Veranda Club.

It was a lot of work making all the arrangements to move from Glens Falls to Florida for the winter, but it was worth the effort. I looked forward to returning the next year. Also, I was happy functioning as a single man and setting a pattern that I was to follow for many years to come.

Chapter 43

I was establishing a new pattern of living with my main residence in Queensbury and spending my winters in Florida.

Before I committed myself to another winter at the Veranda Club, I received a letter from Peter Gagliardi, their very competent manager with whom I had established an excellent relationship. The letter stated that he was now the manager of the Forum in Deerfield Beach, and he encouraged me to apply for winter residence at the Forum. This offer made me very happy, since this had been my first choice the previous year. My sister and her husband checked it out for me and encouraged me to sign the contract. Although the Veranda Club had proven to be very satisfactory, the location of the Forum was better. My sister lived within walking distance, about 2.5 miles, if I chose to get some exercise, since I did not plan to have a car there.

From the winter of 1991-92 through the winter of 2000-01, I returned to Florida gradually increasing my stay to six months. Some of the most important experiences and relationships adding to the quality of my life, after Blossom, would be centered around the Forum.

Living in a retirement residence with about two hundred other aging men and women was a perfect arrangement for my gregarious personality. Also, there was a very capable and friendly staff headed by Peter, and I had an excellent relationship with them. For the first two years before they were fully occupied, I rented a one-bedroom apartment. During this time, I became an important part of the scene lecturing, taking a leadership position in Jewish religious holiday celebrations for the Jewish residents, and actively participating where needed by the activities director in skits and other functions. In the dining room, they gave me the option of floating from table to table rather than sitting with the same people all the time. In this way, I met almost everyone, learned their names, and established relationships. The residents enjoyed my humor and conversation.

With full occupancy and a waiting list, they no longer took part-time residents, but they made an exception for me. When a one-bedroom apartment was no longer available, they offered me a studio apartment that had just been completed. I grabbed it. When this was no longer available, they offered to rent me one of the guest rooms, which was like a large hotel room. Along with this, I would get daily housekeeping and laundry service for my personal articles. They really didn't want to lose me, and I wanted to be there. By being adaptable, it worked out satisfactorily for my future years at the Forum.

My first evening in the dining room was spent with one of the staff. The next evening, I was on my own as I approached the maitre d'. He introduced me to the next man to come along, and we went to our table. This was the beginning of a close friendship that would be stimulating and raise my thoughts to a new, high intellectual level.

He was Dr. Otto L. Bettman, eighty-eight years of age at the time, medium height, with white hair and a white beard and glasses. He bore a resemblance to the great Dr. Sigmund Freud. Because of this, he was invited to play the part of a psychoanalyst in the movie *Lovesick*, filmed in 1981 and featuring Dudley Moore. This was his only movie part, but a new experience in a life full of them. He was very articulate, but he had some accent remaining from his German origin.

Our first meal together was most enjoyable, and I was thrilled at my good fortune in meeting this modest, interesting man, whom I would soon learn was renowned as the founder of the famed Bettman Archive in New York City, one of the world's great picture libraries. He was a widower.

We soon teamed up with two other residents who were well-informed, and the four of us met for dinner very frequently for two winters. Our conversations and sometime arguments covered a wide variety of subjects that were stimulating and interesting. Otto gave our group the name "the Round Table." This was exciting for me because I always had envied the group of intellectuals called the Round Table who met regularly at the Algonquin Hotel in New York City to talk and exchange ideas or the salons in Europe for the same purpose. I had always hungered for more exposure to intellectuals. It was flattering to have a sophisticated New Yorker refer to us in the same manner.

It took a long time to really get to know him and his accomplishments because he did not talk that much about himself. One evening, we got into a discussion about the good old days. These discussions usually nostalgically refer to the greatness of the past when compared to life today. He surprisingly remarked "that the good old days were terrible." When pushed for an explanation, he gave us vivid examples of how sordid life in New York City was a hundred years ago. To our surprise, he then said, "I wrote a book, *The Good Old Days, They Were Terrible.*"

I asked, "Where can I buy the book?" He told me the book was out of print, but he would loan me a copy. When I read it, I appreciated his approach showing how much better off we are today in regard to sanitation, medical care, crime, and even political corruption. At the time, I thought our political and corporate systems were less corrupt, but in 2002, I was not so sure.

The book was well written and full of excellent photographs to go along with the text. I then found out he was the author of fourteen books. The ones I have seen are all replete with illustrations from his famous archive. Since he did not talk about himself very much, I really found out about his many accomplishments by reading his autobiography, *Bettman, the Picture Man.*

Since I was a snowbird, when preparing to leave Florida for the summer, Otto gave me one of his books, *The Delights of Reading,* as a going-away present. This is the inscription dated 4/9/94: "To Orel, my good neighbor (temporarily unfortunately) with warm good wishes and Auf Wiedersehn!" Signed, Otto.

Otto was a very gentle man and gentleman and liked his privacy. Also, he became unhappy with the dining room and decided to make a change. He hired his own cook, and for about the next two years, he was quite reclusive. During this time, I saw very little of him, which was a disappointment, but the best part of our friendship was still to come.

On my return to the Forum in the fall of 1996, I found Otto back in our dining room. He also seemed more comfortable and relaxed in relation to the residents and circulated more than he had in the past. We dined together from time to time, but not on a regular basis. Then, to my surprise, one evening he asked me if just the two of us could dine at a table for two on a regular basis every evening when we were both there. I had always enjoyed being a floater in the dining room, but this appeared to be too good to be true. He seemed very anxious to make the arrangement, and I happily assented.

During the next two winters, we ate most of our dinners together, and for both of us, it was most pleasurable. He knew how to make me feel good by making sure I knew that he had great respect for my background and knowledge. Apparently, from experience, he had the impression that physicians in this country were mostly technicians, and in the past, he had expressed surprise at my intellectual pursuits and knowledge. I think I was a little surprised myself that I could converse on an equal basis about so many subjects with a person with his background and sagacity.

It gave me a sense of accomplishment that a life of study and reading, along with my continued efforts to improve since my retirement, would serve me so well at this time. For example, by joining a Great Books group since retirement, I had read many of the classics of Western and other civilizations that I had no time for during a busy professional and family life. Blossom and I had always been interested in the arts. For many years, I attended the excellent annual lecture program at Skidmore College in Saratoga, "A Survey of Liberal Arts for Mature Adults." I had tried to learn as much as I could about the rich history and traditions of Judaism as well as a smattering of knowledge about other religions. I was a Zionist and was well-informed about the struggle for a Jewish homeland and the wonders and tribulations of the State of Israel. Blossom and I had traveled extensively to many parts of the world and to Israel many times. My interest in gerontology, along with the research in preparing my lectures, had exposed me to a variety of exciting subjects. Also, my humor and jokes were another personal asset.

Our conversations covered many diverse subjects. Otto loved music, was an accomplished pianist, and a Johann Sebastian Bach scholar who wrote two books about Bach. Having been tone deaf all my life, I let him know that probably the biggest gap in my common knowledge was about music, and we didn't discuss it. However, when I told him I was a member of the Phi Beta Kappa Society (an honorary college society in recognition of high attainments in liberal scholarship), he soon presented me with a reprint of an article, "Bach at Potsdam," published in the winter 1982/83 issue of the *American Scholar*. This magazine is published by the Phi Beta Kappa Society and is considered, if not the top, among the top literary magazines in this country.

He was the coauthor of *Pictorial History of American Sports* with John Durant. He wrote in his autobiography, "As for my role, even if I wasn't as beholden to sports as Durant, as a picture maven I knew a good sports shot when I saw it."

He was eager to learn from me about fields where his knowledge was limited, often inquiring about sports and medicine, even though his *The Pictorial History of Medicine* was published in 1956. He was not a world traveler and asked about my travels, and he took a special interest in hearing about Israel in detail.

We also talked about Judaism and the holidays. Although he was not an observant Jew, I thought it would be meaningful if we observed the traditional Friday evening rituals before dinner, Kiddush (prayer over wine), as we shared a small bottle of red wine, and said the Motzi (prayer over challah, the traditional bread). He enjoyed doing this.

He also collaborated with Van Wyck Brooks, whom President Kennedy called "America's first man of letters," on a book, *Our Literary Heritage*, published in 1956. Brooks was impressed by Otto's curiosity and enthusiasm, which also made him such a great companion to be with. Otto also had a wonderful sense of humor brought out in his book *A Word from the Wise* published in 1977, which he describes as . . . a sufficiency of quotes and images to brighten your day. The book is full of wisdom, laughs, and appropriate pictures from cover to cover.

Because of my serious interest in end-of-life-care problems and physician-assisted suicide, we had many interesting discussions about quality and meaning of life and its relation to death. We disagreed in our discussions of many subjects, but our attitudes towards death were very much alike. He was so eloquent in expressing his feelings that I must quote from his autobiography published six years before his death.

Though I have had an interesting and productive life, I have not had my eyes focused on a vita eterna. *Rather, I have tried to condition myself to be always aware of the fragility of life and the limits of our tenure on earth. For me, paradise is simply a poetic fancy rather than a reality I can aspire to. However, I do somewhat envy those who have been blessed with the belief that life on earth is but the prologue to an existence of a higher order. Indeed, I admit I find great appeal in the notion that in the longed-for celestial fields nothing but music fills the air. According to orthodox doctrine, the hosts of angels do not speak, but flutter on "wings of song."*

Nevertheless, tempting as this prospect is, I rather subscribe to Whitman's idea of death as an end "lovely and soothing" or to Henry James's admission of his "fatigue of life" and his wish for the "sweet peace of nothingness." When Freud meditated about his mother's death, he remarked that her demise was a reward for a life well spent. I hope I will be found worthy of a similar gift.

Hence, the prospect of my departure does not cause me tremors of apprehension. Life is a fugue, and like a Bachian fugue, it is predestined to come to its serene, logical, and liberating end.

The dinners with Otto, along with my other activities, made the winter pass too quickly but very happily. When I was departing for the summer, he presented me with another copy of his autobiography, which was inscribed with these words: "To Orel, My friend and ever-spirited dinner companion with every good wish for a pleasant summer, As ever. 4/23/97 Otto"

During the summer, Otto wrote to me and sent me a reprint in color of an article about him in *The Miami Herald* dated July 5, 1997. The following is a small quote from a two-page article: "*Though Bettman could have stopped injecting order into chaos long ago, he did not. At 93, he has just completed a three-year project he calls 'The Eternally Feminine,' a stunning collection of 2,000 photographs and slides of artworks by the masters-Raphael and Rembrandt, Michelangelo and Monet-that feature women as his subject.*

For now, these images are carefully labeled and stored in immaculate files in his study, inaccessible to anyone but Bettman and those he chooses to share them with. He hopes to find someone who will transform this history of women through artwork into a book or put it on a CD-ROM.

'Women are interested in their history,' he says, and 'men are always interested in women.'"

He was a paradigm of gracious mental and physical aging. He wrote me, "And you are generally missed. We are trying to limp along till you return." I was most fortunate to have a wonderful winter home with such friends and family to be with, although Glens Falls was still where I had the stronger roots.

Chapter 44

These winters in Florida were happy and a time of considerable personal advancement physically, mentally, and socially. My activity there in many ways was a continuation of my way of life in Glens Falls.

At the Forum, I lectured frequently to the residents on subjects that interested me at the time and I felt would interest them. In the earlier years, I was passionate about physician-assisted suicide and lectured on this subject to many organizations in and around Glens Falls.

One of the highlights of my speaking career was to be invited to be a guest lecturer in the fall of 1994 "Survey of Liberal Arts for Mature Adults" program at Skidmore College in Saratoga Springs. I had attended this prestigious lecture program given each fall for the aging as a student for many years. I was delighted to serve on the faculty. My subject was "Physician-Assisted Suicide: Is It an Option?" And I even received an honorarium. This course was so popular that each week the same program was given to three different sections of attendees. This required giving the same lecture three days in a row. It was a thrill speaking to my many friends in the section from Warren County where I reside.

Unfortunately, the end-of-life care of that time was abysmal, with people fearing death after a long, painful illness with loss of dignity and control. They said, "I am not afraid to die, but I do not want to suffer." The sad part was they did suffer. I do not believe there is any redemptive value in unnecessary suffering.

On Friday, June 10, 1994, the following interview with me was published in *The Post-Star* under this heading: **Should assisted suicide be an option? Glens Falls doctor says yes, will give talk on subject on Monday. By Jean Trottier, Correspondent.**

With "suicide doctor" Jack Kevorkian frequently making the headlines for his role in helping terminally ill people commit suicide, suicide has heated up. Laws have been passed in several Midwest states hoping to stop Kevorkian, but, according to news reports, the Michigan doctor has supporters and sympathizers. Glens Falls physician Dr. Orel Friedman said he understands what Kevorkian is doing. Although he doesn't advocate physician-assisted suicide, Friedman said he has researched the issue and has come to believe that it should be considered an option for terminally ill people.

He will speak about his opinions on the matter at 1 p.m. Monday at the Greater Glens Falls Senior Center. His talk-"Physician Assisted Suicide-Is It An Option?"-is free and open to the public.

Friedman said his conclusion came out of his professional observations, his personal involvement with friends and family, and his viewpoint of 80 years.

"What is at stake here is the patient's right-to die," he said. "The prolongation of dying and the suffering that goes along with it in our society today is inhuman and insensitive to the desires of terminally ill patients as well as a severe financial drain on their resources and those of the community."

However, he cautioned, physician-assisted suicide should only be considered for the person with no more than six months to live, who is not getting adequate pain control and whose quality of life is poor.

"These people with no hope of recovery have been crying loudly for help for many years and we as an enlightened society supposedly concerned about human rights haven't been listening," he said. "I don't think Dr. Kevorkian is the cause or the solution to the problem, but he has made a definite contribution by making us aware and listen to their cries."

Retired after 30 years as an ear, nose and throat specialist in Glens Falls, Friedman was involved in gerontology for about 10 years after he retired from his practice.

He ran a film series-dispelling the myths and stereotypes of the aged-at Crandall Library for two years and did utilization review for three area nursing homes, determining the classifications of patients and what treatment they required.

Physician assisted suicide was not an issue 50 or 75 years ago, he said. People died at home without the benefit of life support systems that are available to-day. But society has not made similar advances in the psychosocial or ethical approach to the same problems.

"I have heard many people say, 'I don't fear death, but I don't want to suffer,' and under present circumstances many will suffer," Friedman said.

And while death will relieve suffering, it is the final solution.

Many people change their minds when they reach the terminal stage of life and want to hang on despite all the agony, he said.

"Whatever approach we use we have to respect the wishes of the person."

Friedman stressed that there is a difference between physician-assisted suicide and the use of living wills, which designate that no extreme measures of life support will be used, and proxies, which give another person legal power to speak for the dying person, in the issue of death and dying.

"Living wills and proxies have become a very important aspect in the solution," he said. "But even today there are people on life support when for every good reason they should not be."

It has been recommended that a state law be passed that would accommodate the person with no living will or proxy-where a person will be designated to speak for the terminally ill person and decide the course to be followed, Friedman said.

But beyond this the medical, legal and religious communities must get together and pass some type of legislation which will meet the needs of everyone concerned, he added.

Doctors today can take away life support, but they can't actively involve themselves in mercy killing, he said.

"The potential for abuse is real. Any legislation can and must include safeguards against abuse such as the family of a terminally ill person who is a problem to them," Friedman said.

Both doctors and patients are affected by this dilemma-for different reasons.

"I have heard prominent physicians say they believe in giving a person enough morphine (to control pain) even if it hastens death," he said.

However, the prescription a doctor writes for these controlled substances is done in triplicate with a copy going to the Drug Enforcement Agency. The computer may show that he is writing a suspiciously high number of prescriptions when he is just practicing caring medicine, Friedman said.

"The least that can happen is wasting a lot of the doctor's time explaining the circumstances, and the worst is that the doctor could possibly be prosecuted."

When Friedman was talking about this subject last winter to a group of seniors at his retirement community in Florida, a woman related an experience when her husband had been terminally ill.

She told him that there was another patient was dying in the same hospital at the same time. The doctor treating these two patients, the woman said, was afraid to administer enough morphine to both patients to keep them comfortable and hasten death because of the ethical complications.

As a result, she told him, her husband suffered much longer than he should have.

Progress is being made with legislation that will meet the needs of the dying, Friedman said. Both Washington and California have strong grassroots movements that have placed a referendum on the ballots. However, both measures were defeated.

Two groups, Compassion in Dying and the Hemlock Society, assist the terminally ill by providing moral support and information for the terminally ill contemplating suicide, he said.

"Hopefully there will be improvement in pain control of terminally ill patients as in the hospice movement, which will ultimately obviate the need for hastening death in many patients," he said.

"However, those of us who are facing the terminal period of our lives can do so with more equanimity in the near future if a legal solution is found that will safeguard the rights of everyone concerned."

As a result of the publicity, there was a good turnout for my talk, and most of the questions and comments were supportive. However, a couple of days after the above newspaper article appeared, I went to the post office where an aging devout Catholic acquaintance gave me a real calling down regarding my remarks about suffering and physician-assisted suicide. She said something like this: "We have to suffer on this earth if we want to go to heaven." All I could reply was, "You have a perfect right to your ideas, but don't try to impose them on those who have different ones and disagree with you."

In regard to control, the conservatives in America have been able to block most legislation favoring physician-assisted suicide, which I prefer to call physician-assisted death. One breakthrough occurred in the state of Oregon where landmark legislation, although somewhat inadequate, was passed and has been in effect about four years. Only a very limited number of people have chosen to die this way, and to all appearances, the program is a real success. The abuses that the opponents predicted would occur have not occurred.

One of the reasons so few have taken advantage of the program is that the legislation has motivated physicians in Oregon to provide the very highest quality of end-of-life care.

This has been the goal right along to encourage the improvement of care to a degree that the vast majority of dying patients will die pain free and with dignity.

In recent years, I have changed my lectures to take a broader approach, and now the title is, "End-of-Life Care." Progress is being made, hospice has been a positive factor, but we still have a long way to go to reach the goal of people who think as I do.

There is another problem that many will face. For example, what if an aging woman develops dementia, such as Alzheimer's disease, and is in an early-enough stage to know that that she faces a long period of dependency that will be extremely stressful for the family as caregivers and/or prolonged institutionalization. While the victim is still able to make a decision, should she be allowed to decide when and how she should die instead of facing years of impaired physical life while she is mentally and emotionally dead? I think she should have a choice, and family and society should support her decision if she chooses to end her life. As a matter of policy, we are probably not ready for this approach in our society, but enlightened individuals may find a way to act on it. I hope I will have the courage of my convictions if I am faced with a problem of that nature.

Chapter 45

The 1990s were a very productive period when I prepared and lectured on a variety of subjects in addition to end-of-life care.

One of the local organizations asked me to speak about medical care in Israel. It was a labor of love preparing a talk about the health system, and I included the impressions gained from my two stints in the old-age and nursing home in Netanya, Israel. The title of my talk was "Medicine and the Care of the Aging in Israel."

This is the introduction: "*There is a saying, 'That you can judge the quality of life in a country by the way they treat their very young and very old.' I have been to Israel twenty times, and from personal observation, I can tell you that under the circumstances of life there, they do a very good job of taking care of the young and old and also those in between.*" I explained the demographics of the population all of whom, Jew, Arab, or Christian, come under the care of the socialized system that has been the backbone of care since the founding of the state. More recently, health maintenance organizations and a limited amount of private practice have also provided care. The standards are high, with first-rate hospitals providing the best medical care in the Middle East along with excellent medical and dental schools where much scientific research is carried out.

The public health system does a fantastic job dealing with hundreds of thousands of new immigrants, many of whom come from backward countries, like Ethiopia, where malnutrition, tropical and parasitic diseases are rampant. Most of the Russian immigrants have not had any basic immunizations and were accustomed to the practice of abortion for birth control. Despite very difficult circumstances, medical care is available to everyone.

My experience working as a volunteer in the old-age and nursing home for a total of five months was a very positive one. Many of the residents had come to Israel in their later years under the Law of Return, whereby all Jews are admitted regardless of age, physical condition, and finances. Some had never worked in Israel but were afforded the same free care as the other residents. There was a caring, competent staff, and all the basics were provided but no luxuries. The volunteers helped provide nonprofessional services that the limited staff could not always do, like take wheelchair patients out to sit in the sun on nice days.

For those who can afford it, Israel has modern retirement centers comparable to those found in the United States.

I was happy to be able to show that the medical care in Israel is being carried out in a reliable manner under difficult circumstances.

In chapter 27, I described my practice of budgeting. It was no surprise to discover that few of my acquaintances used a budget. Because my simple system served me well, I prepared a talk, "Budgeting for the Retiree," to present to aging groups, which was given several times. It had a good reception, but I doubt that I influenced many of the listeners to undertake the task. A good budget is the underpinning for wise financial planning, and for me, it is no longer a task but something I enjoy doing.

The book *The Fountain of Age*, by Betty Friedan, published in 1993 was the inspiration for another talk I prepared using the book title as its name. This book was used as the starting point of my presentation because Betty Friedan repeatedly expresses her disdain for retirement centers, assisted living facilities, and nursing homes. I do not agree with her in this regard, but it is a good book.

The widespread development of retirement centers in the past two decades is a response to the changing lifestyle requirements of our aging population.

The decision to move from one's home and sometimes one's community to a very different type of residence for the rest of one's life requires much thought and is often difficult.

When I prepared my talk, "The Fountain of Age," it had been my unique experience to spend about six months of the previous five years in community living in my own home in Queensbury and the remainder of the year in a life-care retirement center in

Florida. Life-care is where the facility provides independent living, assisted living, and a nursing home.

Because of my opportunity to experience both lifestyles in the same year over a period of time, my talk compared them on the basis of my subjective feelings and objective observations.

The choices we have to make in our later years are conditioned by factors that are different from those we faced when younger. Age does make a difference. Therefore, we have to be flexible and informed before we make crucial decisions about housing and lifestyles. This talk was designed to provide information and a comparison of the advantages and disadvantages of both community and retirement-center living. I tried to be realistic about the costs involved. At that time, I was happy living both ways, but nothing is forever. When a choice had to be made, it was for an independent-living retirement center in my hometown. Based on my knowledge, the choice was easy.

I had a good response when I gave this talk on several occasions.

I concluded one of my presentations as follows: "*Because of our individual differences, it is beneficial for the aging to have a choice of lifestyles. In the process of life we must make choices based on our present needs, not on fixed ideas of our younger days. If we will it, there can still be fulfillment and a 'Fountain of Age.' And remember, Shakespeare said, 'Our fate lies not in our stars, but in ourselves.'*"

I always laced my many lectures with jokes, which added zest to the talks and always drew a good response from my audiences. My reputation as a humorist was growing rapidly, and several years ago, I decided to prepare a talk entitled "Humor and Aging." My purpose was to overcome the distorted view that the aging are dull, irritable, forgetful, asexual, and inactive physically. Often, jokes contribute to these myths, and if we know what is behind these put-down jokes, we can handle them in a more confident manner by laughing **with** each other and not **at** each other. When these jokes are told by someone in our age group with similar problems and experiences, we should not be offended. However, I would react differently if a twenty-year-old told those same jokes to a group of aging people, or I was the only aging person among a group of young people when those jokes are told. That would be laughing at our age group.

Included in the talk was a presentation of a philosophy, not original with me, that has helped sustain me in the windings and turnings of life—that life is a **process** and not a **possession.**

If we look upon life as a possession, then every transition, even the happy ones, can appear as a loss. For example, getting married can look like a loss of independence. The empty nest means you have lost your children. When parents or spouses die, you feel part of you was buried with them. As possessions, youthful looks and athletic ability do not last forever. The possible losses are endless, and in the course of a lifetime, you may have nothing left but a sense of despair. We know depressed people don't smile very much.

In contrast, when we look upon life as a process and not a possession, marriage, the empty nest, death, change in youthful appearance, and retirement are looked upon as part of the process. As we progress from one stage to another, for a successful transition, **each new beginning must start with an ending.** We cannot straddle fences because this leads to doubt, guilt, and a loss of self-esteem.

I told jokes throughout the talk to illustrate and reinforce the ideas that were being expressed. This proved to be a very successful program.

My desire to approach humor from a different and broader standpoint led to a new lecture, "A Time to Laugh." This title was taken from a line from the famous passage from the book of Ecclesiastes in the scriptures, "a time to weep, and a time to laugh." I talked about how humor works as a positive power in our bodies and lives. I have a wonderful collection of jokes to tell throughout the program and really keep and leave my audience laughing.

How does laughter work? When one laughs, chemicals called **endorphins** are released by the brain that can give you a good feeling, a "high." The endorphins can relieve the sensation of pain, can alter emotional responses and stress, and can have healing effects on our bodies by improving the immune system. They cause the "high" that joggers so enjoy.

I change the jokes from time to time, and this has been a very rewarding program. As much as my audiences enjoy this and my other programs, I feel I am having the best time. It is a labor of love and brings me a great deal of personal satisfaction and pleasure.

Chapter 46

During the summer of 1994, I received a bulletin from my winter residence, the Forum, that stated a class in creative writing was being offered there for the residents to be taught by a professional teacher. This was exciting for me because of my interest in and love for writing. I looked forward to joining the class when I arrived there in the fall but was very disappointed to learn the class had been canceled for lack of interest.

Much to my surprise and joy, when I arrived at the Forum in the fall of 1995, there was an active writer's workshop functioning there. This group had been formed earlier in the year by the residents under the inspired leadership of two newcomers, Leon and Ruth Robinson, a great husband-and-wife team.

Leon's hobby was writing, and his works had been published. Ruth was a capable writer and a superb editor. The following is from the *Deerfield Beach/Lighthouse Point Times*, March 26, 1998:

Leon Robinson started The Writer's Workshop three years ago when he and his wife felt a need for intellectual stimulation within their community. He said, "Our theory is that, if you're having hearing trouble, you get a hearing aid for your ear. And, if you are having trouble with other parts of your body, you can find a remedy. But, for your mind, you need some therapeutic action, a medicine to keep you going over a period of time."

The medicine he came up with was the Writer's Workshop.

I found out that the workshop met every Saturday morning at 10 AM, and I showed up for the class the first Saturday I was there. Leon and Ruth Robinson were strangers to me. They and the group, most of whom I knew, gave me a very warm welcome.

Then I was presented with printed suggestions regarding writing and critiquing and was informed that the meetings started sharply at 10 AM and tardiness was unacceptable. About twelve people were in attendance, which varied slightly over the years.

We soon got down to business when each person present would distribute copies of his or her writing to each one there. Then the writer read what had been written that week, and then each classmate was called upon to critique the article basically using the guidelines that I had just received. Leon Robinson gave the last critique and his impression of the quality of the writing. This process was repeated until everyone, including the Robinsons, had made a presentation.

It was obvious that this was a serious group which was doing good work. One of the requirements was that we write something each week. Leon had a sense of humor, and the participants were having a good time. All this impressed and pleased me with the realization that I would be part of this activity.

However, I was surprised that despite the good quality of the content of the writing, some of the presentations showed poor spelling, sentence structure, and grammar. Nothing was said about these deficiencies in the critiques, which seemed strange to me since I always thought they were important for good writing. Fortunately, I had sense enough in the beginning to observe, listen, and keep my mouth shut, although this approach seemed wrong to me.

Correct spelling, sentence structure, and grammar have been my foundation for good writing all my life. I also insisted that our children follow what to me was the only correct approach. Just to show what a stickler I was when our children left home to go to camp, travel, be exchange and college students, they were instructed where possible to write letters and not call on the telephone. They did write quite often, and the letters were interesting and, for the most part, well written. However, where there were glaring errors in the writing, I acted like a teacher and corrected the errors in spelling and grammar and returned their corrected letters to them. In retrospect, it is remarkable that they were not turned off to the extent that they stopped writing to us. Today, I am kind of ashamed when I think back at what I did, but they all turned out to be excellent letter writers and proficient in the English language in their professional lives and writings.

Needless to say, as I began writing and enjoying the workshop, I gained a great deal from having my work sincerely critiqued, which is the essence of the workshop. One of the lessons which no one had to teach me was not to take negative comments personally. I was constantly irked by the deficiencies in spelling and grammar. After having become well integrated in the group and had their respect, I critiqued a writing, which had excellent content but poor spelling, negatively because of the spelling. Leon strongly admonished me and told me one of the rules was not to critique these errors. This was a rule that he had established in the beginning before I joined the group.

This approach displeased me because I felt the writers could improve if their errors were pointed out. After this episode, Leon and I discussed the matter privately, and he pointed out that most of the class had no previous writing experience and would be turned off if anything other than content was emphasized. I gradually came to accept his point of view, since I could not argue with the success of the endeavor. Perhaps the professional teacher failed to maintain interest in the previous attempt to teach creative writing because the demands were too much for those with limited writing backgrounds. This was an important lesson for me because under the same circumstances, I would have failed as a teacher.

I soon discovered one of the reasons Leon had such insight was because he was poor at spelling despite the fact that he was an excellent writer. Ruth edited his writings to correct the spelling.

My first winter in the workshop was an exhilarating experience. Our group was a family within the Forum family and something special for camaraderie and mutual support. For example, one of the members told us she was depressed and contemplated suicide on coming to the Forum, and the workshop had given her a sense of friendship, worth, and belonging, which drastically improved her mood. We celebrated birthdays together and had an annual banquet in a fine restaurant for our membership. On at least two occasions, we even conducted memorial services.

When spring came, my departure for the summer resulted in stronger feelings of separation from my friends and my activities than I had ever experienced before. This resulted from my attachment to the writer's group. During the summer, I received a copy of the first "Night With the Authors" program in which every member of the Writer's Workshop orally presented one of their original works to a gathering of the Forum family and friends. The program had been well received.

Not long after my return the next winter, Leon informed me that the next "Night With the Authors" would be held in the spring before I left because he and the group wanted me to be its chairman. This was an honor and a big responsibility because this meant participating with Leon and Ruth in the choice of each presentation, along with editing them to be suitable for the author to read. Also, all the papers would be made into a collection that would be presented to each participant and someone we honored like the Forum manager. For this purpose, the writings had to be edited for spelling, grammar, and sentence structure.

Fortunately, when someone presented a real good piece of writing in class, Leon had the foresight to set it aside as a possible choice for presentation. This limited the number of articles and poems we had to review.

Several of our group volunteered to work with me as a committee to plan and make all the arrangements. It was my desire to add humor to an otherwise serious program. I worked very hard preparing a humorous introduction for each speaker that in most cases did not relate to the person's personality. The introductions were finalized working with the committee. The second "Night With the Authors" was a great success, with excellent presentations preceded by an introduction that brought lots of laughs.

One woman was introduced as a bed salesperson who specialized in selling beds to newlyweds. The punch line, "She stands behind every bed she sells," had been picked up listening to Blossom's brothers joking about the furniture business. It went over big, and the person referred to laughed about it for a long time.

Another introduction was something I could not resist since it was a little closer to the author's personality. This came from an old joke about a man who was very successful in the bull-raising business selling bulls all over the world and was known as the biggest "bull shipper" in the country. This brought a lot of laughs, but I apologized to him afterward and never did it again to anyone in the future.

The success of the affair gave me a permanent job as the annual chairman as long as I was at the Forum. However, after a couple of years, I ran out of good humorous introductions and reverted to more conventional ones. This affair was the highlight of the year for the writers and the Forum family.

What was most astounding about these affairs was the demonstration that Leon, Ruth, and the workshop were able to take aging people who had never done any writing and public speaking and mold them into capable writers and confident speakers. It had long been my belief that speakers are made and not born. I now believe the same holds true for writers.

Chapter 47

Just belonging to the Writer's Workshop was one of the best things to happen to me in retirement, but the best was still to come. It was the unbelievable experience of joining with the other twelve members of the class to write a murder mystery novel, *Eighteen by Thirteen*, which was published.

The book was Leon Robinson's brainchild. He surprised us one Saturday when he presented the first chapter that he had written and said, "I challenge you to write a novel based on this first chapter." We all had copies of the first chapter and were told that in two weeks, each of us should present a second chapter based on the first one. In two weeks, we all read our second chapters. It was the custom of the workshop for each member to have a copy to follow as well as to hear so nothing would be missed. After the readings, we decided that since Ruth Robinson was such a superb editor, she should be given the task of picking out the best parts of the various submissions and blend them into a definitive second chapter. Two weeks later, when she presented the second chapter to the group, we knew we were on the right path because it followed the first chapter in a believable, interesting manner.

We followed this same approach every two weeks until we had written sixteen chapters of a murder mystery that included blackmail, love, betrayal, and a close look into the world of crime. At this point, Leon told us we were to conclude our novel with two more chapters.

Writing those last two chapters was a time of inspiration for me. Ideas were flowing through my mind so rapidly that I could not wait to get to my word processor and write. This was the greatest writing experience of my life, and I loved every minute of it. I was convinced these chapters would make a great ending for the story. At first, it was disappointing that the conclusion that was used was not mine, but this passed very quickly. The success of the book proved that the editing and choice of the concluding chapters had been very well done.

It was gratifying that much that I had written was used in the story. The great thing about our book was that the flow appeared as if it had been written by one author. We were seeking a name for our novel, and Leon suggested "Eighteen by Thirteen," representing eighteen chapters by thirteen authors. The title caught on and was a good choice.

The book was finished just before I left for the summer, but the Robinsons kept me informed since we decided to try and get it published. They contacted several publishers, and it became obvious that unknowns like us would have to pay a publisher to do the job. They are in a category called "vanity publishers" and enable people willing to pay to get published. Before submitting the manuscript to anyone, we paid a professional to prepare it in the proper form desired by the publishers.

Art Salzfass, publisher and owner of Rutledge Books in Danbury, Connecticut, agreed to publish our book in paperback for $9,100. In return, we would receive a percentage of each book sold. In an article published in *The Sun-Sentinel* in Florida on July 22, 1998, he was quoted as follows: "*There is an old adage that one of the tragedies of life is to die with your music still in you,*" *Salzfass said.* "*These authors found a way to express their music. They have resonated with one another and we were proud to be a part of that.*"

I missed the discussion in the workshop, but some authors did not want to contribute in order to proceed to publication, but the majority did. The decision was to set up ten shares costing $910, and we could subscribe to a fraction of a share or to one or more shares. I took one share, and all the money was subscribed. Then a "Collaboration Agreement" was drawn up on December 6, 1997, to make our actions legal and protect us. Four writers did not subscribe, and one of the writers who was very enthusiastic about publication bought the most shares. In a very gracious act, she gave each of the four nonsubscribers a 1.25 percent share, worth $113.75, from her own shares so that none of the authors would be left out.

During the winter, we were excited to receive the proofs that we had to edit and approve. No professional proofreader was used by the publisher or by us. We went over the proofs very carefully individually and then collectively decided on the final form which was returned to Rutledge Books. Later on, a proposed cover was sent to us, which was attractive and received our approval. We received word that the book would be out by late spring, and everyone was bursting from anticipation. We were very pleased with our published novel when it was received.

I was back in Glens Falls when plans were made to introduce *Eighteen by Thirteen* to the public at a book signing to be held at the Forum on June 26, 1998. There was considerable advance publicity, which included an agreement made to share the proceeds from the sale with the Alzheimer's Family Center. I made arrangements to fly to Florida to be there with my colleagues on the big day. Shortly before leaving, I received a call from Ruth Robinson telling me that Leon had had a serious heart attack and was in the hospital. She informed me that I was to take Leon's place, chair the event, and make an introductory speech. I agreed.

I arrived at the Forum the afternoon before the signing, which was scheduled for 1:30 PM. When Ruth and I got together, she outlined the planned program and handed me a speech that she had written for me to give because time was so short. Although her intentions were the best, I had never had anyone ghost write a speech for me, and I knew that to make the presentation plausible, I had to prepare it myself even though some of her material could be used. That evening and the next morning, I devoted myself to writing my speech in longhand, since I had no word processor. I just about finished it in time.

The following is from *The Sun-Sentinel*: *"It* was as *close to being a celebrity as 84 year old Orel Friedman had ever been.*

He had just flown in on a red-eye from Albany and people were lining up for his autograph at the Deer Creek Forum in Deerfield Beach. The room had all the glitz and electricity of a Hollywood movie premiere. Cameras clicked, fans eagerly asked questions and accolades gushed forward from each person waiting for a book to be signed.

But Friedman was not alone. He was just one of thirteen authors of the book 'Eighteen by Thirteen,' a mystery written by the Writer's Workshop at the Deer Creek Forum retirement residence."

Further on in the article was the following about me: *"Writing this book was a part of my desire to live every day of my life fully,"* he said. *"This was an experience I'll remember forever."*

Ruth carried out her part of the program very effectively. The authors sat in a line and had a great time signing book after book as they were passed along to us. The signing and sale was a success, and we were a happy, tired group when it was over.

That evening, Ruth and I visited Leon in the hospital, and he appeared very ill. We reported on the events of the day, which cheered him up. I saw my sister Martha at the book signing and enjoyed visiting with my friends at the Forum. The following day, I flew home.

I was on a "high" from this experience, and I decided that my summer would be devoted to publicizing and promoting our novel. The only major bookstore in town was in Aviation Mall, and I worked hard trying to get them to stock our book. However, the headquarters of the chain turned down my request, which upset me since I had no outlet for sales. I had no desire or intention to personally handle sales.

I called Art Salzfass of Rutledge Books, our publisher, who could not help me get our book in the local store. We had a flyer that advertised *Eighteen by Thirteen* for $12.95 plus $3.50 shipping and handling (S&H) to be purchased by calling the publisher's 800 number. He sensed my frustration when I complained that most people would rebel at paying $3.50 for shipping and handling. He saw that I was aggressive, and since he was also anxious to see the book sell, he said, "Anyone who calls to order the book and mentions your name will not be charged for S&H." This made me feel much better and worked very well because this statement was added to the flyer and all the publicity.

I worked diligently and contacted the local newspapers and our local television station for interviews. Excellent articles about the book and me appeared in our local newspapers, *The Chronicle* and *The Post-Star*, and *The Jewish World* published in Albany. Mary Adams was very gracious and interviewed me on channel 8, our local TV station. I wrote articles for the bulletins of several local organizations and the colleges I had attended. All this publicity aroused a great deal of interest in our novel, and I became somewhat of a celebrity. Our publisher told me he was getting telephone orders regularly, and people approached me after reading it with very favorable comments. All my hard work was paying off, and I was having a great summer.

The frosting on the cake was the invitation from *The Chronicle* to participate in their annual book fair on Sunday, October 25, 1998, at Adirondack Community College. I would have to bring a table to set up my books for sale, and I prepared a large poster showing clippings, pictures, and comments about *Eighteen by Thirteen*. They had lectures all afternoon, and I was given a thirty-minute slot. The publicity said, "Dr. Friedman reads from and discusses his book at Adirondack Community College at 2 PM."

Since I had no idea how many books would sell, I ordered a conservative number from the publisher. Also Temple Beth El had a religious book fair the Saturday evening before the Chronicle Book Fair, and as a favor to me, they allowed me to exhibit and sell our book, which sold quite well.

A large, enthusiastic crowd attended the Sunday event, and I had a ball greeting a steady stream of old friends, former patients, and strangers who wanted to talk about the book. Many bought it, and of course, I signed each book. Before too long, I ran out of books and had to tell my customers to order by phone. That would not be the same as a signed copy. Fortunately, I had a large supply of bookmarks with the name of our book and the authors which I gave with each book, and I hit on the idea of signing and giving a bookmark to each person to whom I gave a phone order flyer. This worked out well with no complaints.

It was a long, tiring afternoon, which I enjoyed immensely and paid off. The profits went to our collaborative group and not to me. Since they only supplied space, I had to lug my own table, chair, poster, poster stand, and books to the college and all but the books back to my home. I was invited to participate the next year by Cathy DeDe of *The Chronicle*, but it took place just before I left for Florida for the winter. I just didn't have the energy to prepare for Florida and the book fair at the same time, and regretfully, I declined. However, "the summer and fall of the book," as I think of it, was stimulating, exciting, and unforgettable.

Chapter 48

During the summer of 1998, Leon Robinson, who had recovered from his second bypass operation, informed me that our group might appear on the ABC talk show *Good Morning America*. I thought he was dreaming, but apparently, our publisher knew that ABC was interested in programs featuring positive accomplishments of aging people. He contacted ABC, and they did decide to tape us in Florida for a program. I definitely wanted to be there for the taping when the arrangements were finalized.

The next thing I heard about the taping was a distress call from Leon near the end of August that Ruth had been taken ill and would not be able to be the leader in the program as had been planned. He intended to participate on a limited basis since he was still quite weak. When the producer of *Good Morning America* found out about Ruth's illness, he threatened to cancel the program, fearing the lack of dynamic leadership. Leon told him about me and his confidence in my ability to handle the job. ABC agreed to put everything on hold until I contacted them. Leon asked me if I would do it, and I was happy to agree, since this was very important for all of us.

My first call was to the associate producer in New York City, and I turned on all my powers of persuasion to show him that I was articulate and experienced as an organizer, leader, and chairman since they had public appearances planned for taping. I impressed him sufficiently to have him suggest that I should speak to his boss, the producer. I was able to reach him a couple of days later, and after our conversation, he agreed to proceed with the taping on September 17 and 18, 1998.

Before completing the call, I told him I would have to fly to Florida from Glens Falls for the taping and asked to have ABC pay my expenses. He agreed to this. I thanked him and then called Leon to give him the good news.

On September 16, I flew to Florida and checked in to a guest room at the Forum. I found out that our program would begin at the First Presbyterian Church in Fort Lauderdale, where we would talk for about one hour to their senior's group about the Writer's Workshop—how it was formed, the problems we faced, writing our book, and how they could start their own group. The room was large and set up with tables for lunch with at least one hundred people in attendance. I was the chairman who introduced the speakers from our group, with Leon speaking first. It went well, and our program was enthusiastically received.

Then we spread out to sit with our hosts for lunch. The conversation was animated, and it was fun. Also there was a table set up for the sale of *Eighteen by Thirteen*. ABC arranged everything and directed the taping of the program.

After lunch, we returned to the Forum, where lights had been set up for taping interviews with the individual members of the workshop during the rest of the afternoon. Tired but happy, we looked forward to the next day.

On Friday morning, September 18, we were taped carrying out our usual daily activities. I was asked to appear outside in the beautiful garden surrounding the Forum swimming pool where I made a walking entrance and then sat on a bench and conversed with residents passing by.

We also set up a bridge table where I was one of four authors to appear like we were playing bridge.

After lunch, we were taped as we carried out the weekly meeting of the Writer's Workshop, which was held a day in advance to accommodate to the producer's schedule. By this time, we were accustomed to the taping and were relaxed. All went well.

Then we waited for the highlight of the program, being interviewed by the host of *Good Morning America*, Kevin Newman. We were told that right after he completed the morning show in New York City, he would fly to Florida and be at the Forum around 3 PM. He was a little late arriving, and we saw him immediately go into a huddle with the producer while we waited. After about thirty minutes, we were asked to take our seats for the taping. Lights had been set up all around, making it look like a movie set.

As he approached us, I was impressed by his physique. He was wearing a shirt open at the collar and a suit, and he appeared to me to have the neck and shoulders of a well-developed athlete. He had appeared slimmer to me when previously watching his program on television. His facial appearance was as expected, handsome and wearing glasses.

He seated himself comfortably in front of us, smiled, and spoke to us in a confident, relaxed manner, which set the tone for the interview. He informed us that he had scanned and partially read *Eighteen by Thirteen* and was impressed. He gave us some instructions and then said in a soothing voice, "Don't worry if you make a mistake because we can just cut it out." As an experienced interviewer, he knew how to make us feel very comfortable before starting the actual taping.

The interview went quite smoothly, and we had a good time. However, when it was over, Leon and many of the others were exhausted. We were running late for a scheduled book signing at Borders Bookstore in Boca Raton, the final event on the taping schedule. So few felt up to any more activity that the book signing was canceled even though we anticipated selling quite a few books.

John Fisher and I spoke to Kevin Newman about his schedule, and he told us he would be leaving later in the evening. This enabled us to invite him to have dinner with us in the Forum dining room. He was friendly, bright, easy to talk to, and interesting. It was an enjoyable experience, and we saw what it is like to be a celebrity since residents kept coming over to greet him. He took all the interruptions in stride and never appeared disturbed. It was a day to remember.

The ABC staff informed us that they would edit the tapings and let us know well in advance when we would appear on *Good Morning America*. During October and November, there was no word from ABC. We began to wonder if our program would ever be shown. Then, one evening in early December, we received a message while having dinner that we would be shown on *Good*

Morning America at 8 AM the next day. I had promised many family members and friends that I would let them know when they could see our program, and I and others were annoyed at ABC's lack of consideration for us. I knew I had to make a lot of phone calls, and my problem was compounded by the fact that I was scheduled to play bridge after dinner, which would keep me away from the telephone for a few hours. I didn't ask to cancel the game, just that we cut it short. My friends were very agreeable, and, before it was too late, I was able to make some calls. I asked those I called to tell others, and many were notified. I waited until the end to call those on the West Coast because it was still early for them.

ABC lost out by not informing us in advance because we could have arranged for newspaper articles about the show in Florida and Glens Falls, which would have increased the number of viewers considerably.

It was exciting watching the actual program. After two days of taping, we were given about a little more than five minutes on television, but it was impressive. All the comments were favorable, and it was an experience to be long remembered.

From time to time over the next two years, we all received royalty checks from our publisher from the continued sale of our book. Just the idea of receiving these checks gave me great satisfaction, since it was further proof of our success as published writers. The royalties never came close to equaling the initial investment with the publisher, but this was not unexpected or important from my standpoint.

During the winter of 1990-91, we were informed by Rutledge Books that they were closing out the sale of *Eighteen by Thirteen*. We were given the opportunity to purchase as many of the remaining books as we wished at a low price. Several of us bought a supply of books. I still have some and give them away as gifts.

Joining twelve colleagues in the creative effort of writing a published, very favorably accepted murder-mystery novel along with collateral publicity, book signings, participating in book fairs, and an appearance on a national television program was a highlight of my intellectual and personal advancement in retirement.

Chapter 49

Judaism and being part of a Jewish community has been an important part of my life both before and in retirement and as a widower.

My childhood exposure to Orthodox Judaism in our synagogue on Jay Street, which blindly followed the Eastern European model based on ignorance and superstition really turned me off. This did not affect my strong acceptance of myself as a member of a Jewish peoplehood, although my first allegiance is as an American. My early religious education left me almost completely ignorant of the rich history, traditions, and culture of my heritage. I wanted and had a bar mitzvah at age thirteen, but instead of being an enjoyable, meaningful rite of passage, it was a negative experience.

My family observed the major Jewish holidays. After becoming established in Schroon Lake, my parents would vacation after the summer season by taking us to Scaroon Manor, a fine hotel nearby where they held High Holiday services. On Passover, we would spend the holiday as a vacation in a kosher hotel in Saratoga. These festive holidays represented my main religious observance during my years of preparation for a medical career. Our college fraternities were segregated, and I belonged to a Jewish fraternity. Most of my friends during those years were Jewish. In the army at Camp Lee, Virginia, there were religious services, and I attended at times because of the fellowship and salami sandwiches that were served afterward.

Blossom grew up in Conservative Judaism in Lebanon, Pennsylvania. Her religious knowledge was also limited. We were in agreement that we would join a liberal congregation rather than a traditional one based on the Eastern European model. When we settled in Glens Falls, we joined the Reform congregation, Temple Beth El, where Kurt Metzger was the Rabbi. We explained to my parents why we were going to make this choice and attend a house of worship different from theirs, and they were very understanding. It never affected our close, loving relationship.

Rabbi Metzger and I became good friends and had many private conversations, where I picked his brain for information. We had no adult education program in our temple in those days, but this was the beginning of my Jewish education. Over the years, Blossom and I gradually accumulated information and knowledge, and we also learned a great deal from our more traditionally observant children. We helped them obtain a much better grounding in Judaism than we ever had by sending them to Jewish camps sponsored by the Reform movement and on programs in Israel. Barbara and Victor attended Brandeis University where she majored in Near East and Judaic studies and Victor majored in Mediterranean studies. His spirituality led him to participate in all phases of Jewish religious observance, and he even attended a yeshiva (a religious school) for one year. Barbara and Beverly both married men who were practicing Orthodox Jews.

Because of the effort we made to improve our Jewish education, we were considered very knowledgeable by most of the congregation.

After Blossom's death, I spent my winters at the Forum in Florida, where there were many Jewish residents, including Dolly and Saul Brivic, who were interested in observing our religious holidays. I offered to cooperate with them, and we made a modest beginning. I decided to take the responsibility for conducting a real Passover Seder on March 5, 1993, to which all the residents of the Forum would be invited. Our manager, Peter Gaglardi, was very pleased with my plans and offered complete cooperation from the activities, dining room, and housekeeping staffs.

Unfortunately, our well-appointed dining room on the second floor was broken up into sections and did not lend itself to a community Seder. I decided to conduct the Seder in our large activities room on the first floor. Logistically, this meant modifying the service in order to complete the Seder without the customary break for the special dinner in the traditional manner. Because the attention span of our residents was limited, I decided to shorten the Seder to one hour and complete it in time to enable the residents who ate at the first seating to get there without rushing.

I assumed all the responsibility for the planning and the arrangements working with the staff. There are hundreds of different Haggadahs that tell the story of Passover for the Seder. I took four of them apart and blended them into our own Haggadah, which included all the most important parts of the story. I timed it for one hour, and in practice, the timing proved accurate.

Then in writing and verbally, I informed the food staff just what ceremonial foods and wine would be needed for the Seder, how to prepare it, and how to serve it, since this was mostly new to them. We worked with housekeeping and the activities director on the table arrangements and flowers. Dolly, the food manager, and I worked out the menu for the Passover-type dinner in the dining room following the Seder.

The story of Passover in the Haggadah lends itself well to be divided into parts so that many readers can participate. I cornered residents, both Jewish and gentile, whom I thought would make good readers, and about fifteen agreed to participate.

The Seder is enhanced by the group singing of several songs. My good friend John Fisher was happy to lead the singing. He has perfect pitch, knows all the songs and the music, and took complete charge of the musical program.

The day of the Seder rolled around. All the hard work paid off. We had a large attendance. For the most part, everything went smoothly, and the comments were favorable. The Seder became a tradition and was looked forward to by the residents every Passover. I didn't return to Florida again after the last one I led in 2001, which was attended by an enthusiastic overflow crowd of more than one hundred. I received many compliments that this was the best Seder I had conducted.

Most of the Seder was conducted in English, and the Hebrew blessings and readings were all translated into English. As a result, several of the Jewish residents told me this was the first time in their lives they understood what the Seder was all about, the story of the Exodus. This made me very happy because this mirrored the ignorance and frustration of my early years when the Hebrew text was never explained or understood.

Conducting these Seders represented to me the second most important accomplishment during my winters at the Forum. The first was taking an important part in the Writer's Workshop and improving my writing skills.

I was involved in our Chanukah and Purim celebrations, but the leadership role was assumed by Ralph Bartel. He developed the Chanukah program and the singing. In the later years, I heard about a program like ours where everyone attending was encouraged to provide his or her menorah so we could carry out the traditional lighting of the candles and saying the blessings together. I suggested this to Ralph, and he thought it was a great idea. We tried this communal approach, and it was very successful and became traditional.

For a few years, Grace Marks was a resident. She wrote a play depicting the Purim story. Ralph Bartel was delighted to have us put on the play for our Purim celebration for a couple of years. Under Grace's direction, we practiced and performed the play with dancing girls, elaborate costumes, and creative props. It was a great success, and we also got some unplanned laughs when Haman, played by one of our oldest residents, bowed before me, King Ahasuerus, and couldn't get up. We had to lift him off the floor, but it was all in fun.

I think we performed the play twice. Then Grace left to move closer to her family, and we were unable to carry on without her and discontinued the performances.

It was fun being involved in these activities, and my religious knowledge was enhanced, which added to the satisfaction I was experiencing in life.

After Blossom's death, I continued to attend services regularly at Temple Beth El and participate in temple social activities when I was in Glens Falls. My attachment to our religious community has been an important part of my life, and I have made friends with the newer, younger members. I feel very close to our Rabbi and his wife, Elaine, and am very comfortable in the temple even though few of my contemporaries are still active. I never spend holiday dinners alone because the Sobels always invite me to their home for a delicious meal and an enjoyable time. I am happy and benefiting from my long association with our religious community and taking advantage of what it has to offer.

Chapter 50

Prior to my departure for the summer, my friend Otto Bettman gave me another copy of his autobiography, *Bettman, the Picture Man*. He signed it: "To Orel, my friend and ever-spirited dinner companion with every good wish for a pleasant summer. As ever. 4/23/97. Otto."

When I returned to the Forum in the fall of 1997 and began dining with my friend Otto, it was obvious that his health was deteriorating. While I was away, he had an accident resulting in a fall. While not life threatening, his injuries started this unusually healthy ninety-three-year-old man on a downward path.

His mind was very clear, and we resumed our close relationship and discussions. Our daily dinners continued to be highlighted by lively and interesting conversation. During the winter, he used a walker and then a wheelchair, and aides were in constant attendance.

For a New Year's present, Otto presented me with a copy of his book *The Delights of Reading* with the inscription,

> "To Orel
> in the hope that some
> of the sayings here presented
> will come in handy to a man
> who himself has stored up
> much wisdom in a long
> and meritorious life.
>
> The Best for '98
> As ever
> 12/31/97   Otto."

He always took great interest in my trips to Israel and was eager for information about the Jewish homeland which he had never visited. In April 1998, I was leaving for a visit to Israel, and he wanted to give me a going-away present. He presented me with a used copy of his book *A Word from the Wise*, published in 1977 and probably out of print. I was flattered since this had to be one of his personal copies and was inscribed, "To my friend and ever spirited table companion Orel with all good wishes for a '98 pilgrimage to Israel . . . and a safe return. 4/10/98 Otto."

Israel was celebrating fifty years of statehood in 1998, and in commemoration of this important event, several outstanding books containing excellent photographs had been published. This was my chance to reciprocate to Otto for the books he had given me, and while in Israel, I sought out and found the best book available in English as a gift for him. I cannot remember the inscription I wrote, but it was appropriate and with much affection for Otto.

My visit with my family there was most enjoyable, and I returned to the Forum bearing my gift which I was anxious to present to my dear friend. To my consternation, I was informed that Otto was quite ill, no longer was coming to the dining room, and was not having visitors.

I called his apartment and spoke to one of his attendants and told her that I had a gift to present to Otto, and I would make my visit brief. After checking with him, she told me he wanted me to come.

He was sitting in a comfortable chair and appeared much weaker than when I saw him before leaving on my trip.

After exchanging warm greetings, I presented him with the book I had brought from Israel as a gift from me. He thanked me and appeared very pleased. We spoke briefly, and I excused myself in keeping with my promise to limit my visit.

The next news about my friend was that he had been hospitalized and was not having visitors. Since I was leaving for the summer in a few days, I called his granddaughter who was in charge and asked if I could see him before I left. She called back and gave me permission.

Visiting a severely ill person can be stressful, but this call turned out to be a pleasant experience. Otto was weak and confined to bed with an intravenous tube in his arm, but his mind was clear. He immediately directed the conversation away from himself and told me how much he appreciated my gift of the book I had given him. He was very impressed with the photographs but had not been able to read much of the text. He wanted to know all about my trip to Israel and what was happening there. The time passed quickly and pleasantly. It was time for farewells, and I left.

I walked out of his room with mixed emotions. He appeared to be in a state of acceptance for what was to come, and this rubbed off on me. However, the knowledge that I might never see or talk to him again was saddening.

Since my departure for the summer was near, I was occupied with packing and other arrangements for my departure on Saturday morning, which was about four days after my visit to the hospital. After dinner Friday, May 1, 1998, the residents of the Forum were informed that Otto had died that day. There was no information about any funeral arrangements, and I had no choice but to sorrowfully leave the next morning as planned.

I watched *The New York Times* for an obituary, and on May 4, an extensive obituary occupying almost half of a page was found. It said: "A private funeral for family and close friends was being planned."

He was in my thoughts during the summer, and I was determined to present a talk in his memory after returning to the Forum in the fall of 1998. Ingrid, our activities director, did a great job photographing the pictures from his autobiography to be projected to illustrate my presentation. My desire was to talk about the man I knew as a person rather than just repeat material available in his autobiography. My efforts paid off when the program was presented because it kept the large audience in rapt attention, and I received many compliments after my talk was over. This would be my final tribute to my dear friend and mentor who enriched my life for seven years during the 1990s with intellectual stimulation and meaningful conversation. I miss him, think of him often, and reread parts of his books from time to time.

Otto was a shining example of Germany's loss and America's gain as a result of Hitler's anti-Semitism, which led many great intellectuals, scientists, and physicians to emigrate from their homeland to save their lives. That is how the great or greatest "picture man" of his time had the opportunity to establish the Bettman Archive and make his contribution to society in the United States instead of the land of his birth.

Because of our many conversations about end-of-life care, it is my belief that Otto was in control until the end and chose the time and manner of his passing. It was a fitting reward for a life well lived.

Chapter 51

At the Forum in 1999, the Writer's Workshop was functioning well with Leon leading the way, but Ruth never was able to function as capably as in the past. The following winter 1999-2000 revealed considerable deterioration in the health of both of them, but we continued our activities with John Dales assuming more responsibility.

John had moved into the Forum a few years previously and, due to my urging, joined the workshop. He showed excellent writing skills, was well organized, and diligent. We worked together well.

The summer of 2000 was another turning point in my life. Joan Stegman, my longtime housekeeper and friend, became ill and required surgery. For a considerable time during the summer, I was without Joan's weekly assistance with the housekeeping and laundry. When she recovered, she knew it would not be possible to provide the same level of help as in the past. During her illness, the quality of my life suffered when I had to do housekeeping and laundry. This was a wake-up call telling me that without her assistance, something had to change.

Fortunately, a senior retirement community was being planned to be built in the Hiland Park area of Queensbury. In the past, out of curiosity, I had looked at the model apartment and their literature in the sales office. Now it dawned on me that this community might be the long-term solution to my problem of living without Joan's help. I investigated it carefully and was impressed by what was being offered.

I decided to sell my house the following year and move to an independent-living retirement center and reside in my new home throughout the year. Where to settle was the problem. I preferred the Florida climate to that of Queensbury, and at the Forum residence, I had many friends and was happy and comfortable there. In Florida, my sister lived nearby, as did Moe and Janet in the winter. We enjoyed getting together.

However, my observations over the years had convinced me that when the aging become dependent, the best place to locate is near their caring child or children if they have them. I had advocated this in my lectures on end-of-life care. Since my very caring daughter Barbara lives in New York City while Beverly and Victor, for all their caring, reside in Israel, I felt that I wanted to be near Barbara. This ruled out Florida. I checked out residences in the New York area and visited a couple. With my background and experience, I knew that I would not be happy residing in them.

The best compromise was to remain in Queensbury and reside in the planned Glen at Hiland Meadows. The area had been my home for most of my life, and the associations were here that had made my life happy. I asked Barbara to come here for a weekend to see what I had in mind, and she enthusiastically approved of my plans. She felt it was close enough to New York for her to provide support if needed and for me to take a bus to New York to visit them. She helped me pick out colors for carpeting and cabinets so I would be all set when I signed up the following week. It was necessary to make the arrangements quickly because it was almost time to leave for Florida, but it was a carefully considered decision.

Joan Stegman, my housekeeper, knew about my plans, and when they were finalized, she was pleased because of her sincere concern for my welfare. She offered to help me in my new home when the time came, and this pleased me because she would be needed but on a more limited basis. Other members of my family were informed of my plans.

I knew it would be traumatic telling my sister and my friends in Florida, especially those in the Writer's Workshop and my golfing companions, of my decision not to winter in Florida in the future. They were surprised, but after explaining my motivation and plans, they flattered me with sincere kind remarks and how much I would be missed.

Leon Robinson's health had deteriorated markedly, and he suffered severe pain and breathing difficulty. He worked at his writing and conducting the workshop almost to the day of his death in the spring of 2001. His wife, Ruth, was too dependent to live alone and wisely moved to Connecticut to live with her daughter there. Their loss was the end of an extremely important era for us. However, the solid foundation they established for the Writer's Workshop has enabled it to function well to this day under the leadership of John Dales.

My contact with the workshop has been maintained since I left, especially because of the writing of this book. It was started at the Forum, and the early chapters were critiqued at the weekly meetings of the workshop. When I left, John Fisher and John Dales, representing the group, said they would appreciate receiving future chapters because they were interested in and enjoying my life story. Also, they would continue to critique my work if I wanted this done. This has worked very well, and I greatly appreciate their input.

I receive their contemporary writings in their bulletins and the proceedings of "The Night With the Authors." The writings are of high quality with my friends John Dales, John Fisher, Jen Maltzman, Julia Nyfield, and, until recently, Doris Bissette, among others including new members contributing regularly. I greatly enjoy the continued relationship.

The summer of 2001 was spent preparing for my move to the soon-to-be completed Glen at Hiland Meadows. Fortunately, I am not weighed down by excessive sentiment that would prevent me from letting go of "things," and I tossed away and tossed away the accumulation of papers, records, and memorabilia of a lifetime. Family was given first choice of furniture and furnishings that I could not use. What they could not take was given away for charitable purposes. I discovered it was a waste of time trying to sell my things since they were not antiques. A large collection of family photographs were passed on to my children.

Fortunately, my home was sold quickly by me as the result of a stroke of luck. I had three very friendly neighbors whom I didn't want to be surprised to see a real estate sign in front of my home. So I told each one of them individually of my plans to move and my intent to engage a real estate firm to sell my house. A few days later, one of these neighbors sent me a customer who bought the house.

The move was made on Friday, November 2, 2001. This date was chosen because Victor had informed me that he was coming from Israel to America for a conference around that time, and he wanted to help me move. Barbara made plans to come from New York with him that afternoon.

In preparation for furnishing my apartment, careful measurements of the floor plan, the wall space, and closet space enabled me to bring the exact amount of furniture, wall hangings, towels, linens, kitchen equipment, dishes, and appliances that I would need without being overcrowded. The easy part was having the movers pack everything, but they had warned me they did not unpack. Unpacking would be the hard part. The move was on Friday morning. Victor and Barbara arrived Friday afternoon and went right to work. By the time they left on Sunday, everything was put away, and not a single carton was left in the apartment. The wall hangings were all in the proper location for the maintenance staff to hang as soon as possible. I was comfortably set from the very beginning. My children did a tremendous job for which I am most appreciative and grateful. Doing all this myself would have taken weeks and be exhausting.

Having lived this lifestyle in Florida for many winters gave me a great deal of insight on how to make the move. Most people bring too much and have no place to put it. As a result, their apartments are cluttered and even uncomfortable for a long time.

I am very happy at the Glen at Hiland Meadows. I have adapted to the cold winter weather and often go out walking when it is not too cold. I am comfortable and have peace of mind. My children also have peace of mind knowing that all is well with me.

Chapter 52

It is almost twenty-five years since my sudden, forced, unplanned retirement from an active practice as an ear, nose, and throat specialist and surgeon because of the abrupt onset of double vision. This disability and the impossibility of immediately obtaining a competent specialist to carry on my practice left me with the choice of practicing as an impaired physician or retiring completely. I chose to retire rather than think about doing anything to harm the welfare of my patients. Also, under no circumstances would I chance ruining my excellent professional reputation. I have always prided myself with the knowledge of when to let go, and although it would be traumatic, the inevitable time had arrived.

My dilemma is described in the earlier chapters, and part 2 shows that the way I left this low point in my life to find happiness, growth as a personality, and fulfillment has been an intellectual and spiritual journey which evolved gradually over the years.

Medicine has been described as a good mistress and a poor master because many physicians have obsessive-compulsive personalities and find their profession all consuming. When all one's self-esteem results from your work, letting go may be extremely difficult, if not impossible psychologically. Total disengagement from medicine with no satisfying replacement can be devastating. Fortunately for me, my dedication to my patients was balanced by a caring, understanding wife and involvement in outside interests and activities. It is fair to consider that medicine was more a mistress than a master in the conduct of my life. Nevertheless, sudden retirement left a void in my life that had to be filled.

This is a regular scenario in an anticipated retirement. Often the first six months to a year finds the male retiree enjoying a so-called honeymoon resulting from a release from the daily grind and using his time catching up on projects in and around the house. Sooner or later, things are taken care of, and if no planning for the use of leisure time has been done, his lack of a structured life and boredom may lead to depression. He becomes irritable, annoys his wife to the point of conflict, and he may start drinking.

Although my busy, structured lifestyle as a physician ended almost overnight, being stuck with a drastic drop in income, an expensive home-office, a hopefully salable medical practice and equipment put me in the same category as the retiree on a honeymoon. I threw much of my energy into an attempt to dispose of this "albatross" to hopefully make my life and finances more comfortable. Despite my diligence by the end of 1980, eight months later, there was nothing to show for my efforts. This was the lowest point of the experience and the closest to becoming depressed. It was at this time that I made the crucial decision to enter the field of gerontology. This did not diminish my dedication to disposing of my unneeded assets.

My career as a gerontologist never brought me any significant financial gain that had been my hope in the beginning, but it brought a foundation upon which the rest of my life has benefited. Blossom and I would undoubtedly have had a successful retirement, but the insight both of us gained in studying the field of aging was a distinct added advantage.

In the next couple of years, my medical equipment was sold, and the home-office was sold after being on the market for five years. I took a considerable loss, but we managed to survive and enjoy life.

Gerontology was the reason for my entrance into becoming an effective and sought-after public speaker. Since I had to prepare all my presentations, my writing and research skills were honed. I was available as a resource person. My interest in observing the everyday life of the aging in differing milieu over the years served as a valuable learning experience. I enjoy being a perpetual student.

As time passed, my love for jokes and stories led me into becoming a recognized humorist. All the laughing has probably strengthened my immune system and protected my health and sense of well-being.

For the first ten years of retirement, Blossom and I traveled extensively and had a wonderful time. After her death, I spent my winters in Florida and visited Israel frequently. Even though I traveled alone, I greatly enjoyed a cruise and tour in Alaska and a tour of the Yellowstone National Park area.

In my life after medicine, I was able to divest myself of inhibitions that kept me more or less politically correct during my years of practice and be myself. It is a wonderful feeling not to have to weigh everything you do or say in order not to appear offensive or unstable. Becoming more objective about matters related to medicine has enabled me to see and evaluate the deficiencies as well as the virtues of the great system which developed in our lifetimes.

Probably the one subject about which I have been a zealous advocate is in the field of end-of-life care. About fifteen years ago, when I first came to recognize and accept how abysmal the care of the dying was in the United States, my energy was invested in lecturing and promoting physician-assisted suicide or (as I prefer it) physician-assisted death. The publicity resulting from Dr. Kevorkian's efforts in this field was a wake-up call that started the improvements we see today. After a while, my lectures were broadened in scope to the wider field of end-of-life care as a vehicle to inform the public on how to have their rights and wishes respected when confronted by insensitive and uncooperative physicians and hospitals. Good progress has been made in recent years, but there is still much room for improvement.

Although strongly supportive of a woman's right to choose how she conducts her reproductive life, I have not been active in this field. However, my observations over the years have convinced me that many men, including male physicians, do not understand female psychology and physiology, even though it is mostly men passing the laws and making the rules that control women's reproductive rights. The Supreme Court's decision on *Rowe v. Wade,* giving a woman the right to choose regarding abortion was a great advance, and I hope it is never overturned.

Religion is an important part of my life and is a significant factor in my spiritual growth in my later years.

Rabbi Richard J. Sobel of Temple Beth El has influenced my religious life in many ways through adult-education classes and workshops, services, and discussions of Torah (the Jewish Scriptures often misnamed the Old Testament), community service such as his leading the annual Hometown Thanksgiving, and our close friendship. Sunny Buchman's spiritual-journey program has added to my knowledge. My children and their families have taught me much about a more traditional Jewish lifestyle than my familiar Reform.

My attachment to Temple Beth El results from a comfortable sense of belonging to a community where we share a feeling of closeness. Worship for me is more rational than emotional. Spirituality for me is not primarily ritualistic, but the manner in which I conduct my daily life. In one of our workshops, we prepared "Ethical Wills," a valuable exercise in actually writing down your principles of conduct to pass on to your heirs. My life since retirement has been enriched by the opportunity to improve to some degree my knowledge of the rich tradition, practices, and culture of Judaism and the forces that shaped our history. I have gained enough understanding to comfortably approach Judaism from a liberal rather a fundamentalist standpoint.

My problem with fundamentalism in any religious group is that generally the fundamentalists consider their viewpoint the only acceptable one. There is no tolerance for any other approach to religion or human conduct but theirs. History records all kinds of atrocities carried out in support of their zealotry, and we see it today.

What troubles me at present is the trend to use religious beliefs to try to set the standards and interfere in the personal lives and actions of the general public who disagree with them. If any individual's or group's religious beliefs make abortion, family planning, physician-assisted death and differing sexual orientation unacceptable to them, they have every right to act on them for themselves. However, the very same individuals and groups have no right to try to impose their beliefs, no matter how sincere, on those of us who approach life from a different viewpoint. I do not believe that there is any redemptive value in terminal suffering, and no one has the right to make me think or act differently. Separation of church and state has made America great, and I believe that those who are trying to break down those barriers of separation are acting to the detriment of our great nation.

Time has taken its toll on most of my close friendships, but my life is still enriched by many new friendships even though they are not the close ones of yesteryear mainly because we do not spend very much time together. It has been my good fortune to make the acquaintance of younger people with common interests, and we have become friends. Also, I know many people from the weekly duplicate bridge game at the senior center, golf at the country club, the Glens Falls Association for the Hearing Impaired and its bridge group, our Great Books study group, and our temple and synagogue in Glens Falls. Retiring and remaining in my hometown gives me the pleasure of running into former hospital and professional associates, as well as former patients and chatting with them. One of the important benefits of living in a retirement center is the interpersonal relationships that can be quickly established. I still am in touch with some of my Florida friends from the Forum where I lived for many winters. This is my good fortune.

Nothing can take place of a loving, caring family, which is a blessing that I have been privileged to enjoy all my life starting with my parents and their contemporaries. There has always been a close, friendly relationship with my sister and brother and their families. Our in-laws and their friends and families became our friends. As an example, out of the goodness of their hearts, Moe and Janet Friedman threw a birthday party for Lilli Seligson, our daughter Beverly's mother-in-law, from Finland, at their camp on Schroon Lake. All of Lilli's numerous relatives in the United States and Canada were invited, and many came. The party went on for about four days, and everybody had a great time in a delightful setting, great food, and socializing, all hosted by Moe and Janet.

Our large extended family tries to maintain contact and visit as frequently as possible and have lots of parties. Blossom came from a big family that scattered all over the United States. When the family all came together for some kind of a party, it appeared like a convention. Having two families living in Israel does not result in as close a relationship with my grandchildren as I would like. But we visit back and forth often enough to have a loving relationship.

My interest in end-of-life care is more than academic. Many aging people say, "I do not fear death, but I do not want to suffer." I confess I fear death at this time. Even at the age of ninety-one, I do not want to face up to my mortality because I am enjoying life. My fear results from not wanting to terminate a good life. When my lifestyle makes the probable change to disability and suffering, then I hope I will not fear death but accept it as a reward for a life well lived.

Jewish theology does not emphasize an afterlife. It is my belief that our conduct in our lifetime determines to a great degree whether our lives on earth will be "heaven" or "hell." The quality of my life on earth is the only heaven or hell that concerns me. However, because there are happenings beyond our control, our goals may not be met. We also know that good is not always rewarded, and evil is not always punished. If the ethical principles I practice and the activities I engage in set a desirable example for my progeny and, possibly, society to use as guidelines in their lives, this to me will be my afterlife or immortality.

Most of us have a dual existence. First, there is a personal and family world, and the other relates to people and happenings in our country, events in foreign societies and cultures and outer space.

An important part of our inner or personal life is related to family, friends, our day-to-day existence, and the life cycle events from birth to death. This is the keystone on which our worldly heaven or hell or something in between is built. Given a good foundation, those who work at it and are fortunate can find an inner world of equanimity and peace as a shelter when buffeted by the storms of the outer world over which we may not have control.

What are these storms? Despite the fantastic technological and medical advances seen in my lifetime, in the world around us, there is war not peace, terrorism is a constant threat, disease and hunger plague much of our world population. The worst sins in facing all these problems are indifference and a defeatist attitude that, as individuals, we have can have no influence on what is happening. A glaring example is that large share of the population who do not vote in elections saying their vote or votes do not count. We must be concerned and involved, but our efforts should not lead to zealotry, "where the cure is worse than the disease."

Passion and hard work for the causes we believe in is important. But for good physical and mental health, there has to be an inner, personal world to retreat to for support and to escape from the pressures, disappointments, and negative occurrences on the outside.

Twenty-five years after a forced retirement from the practice of medicine and a bleak period in my life, my review of these years puts me in an exhilarating positive mood. Had I been able to continue in my practice and planned my future retirement, there would not have been the motivation and incentive to become the person that I know I am. Nor in all humility would I have gained the respect and admiration with which others look upon me and my life. Yes, there is a life after medicine, and it can be satisfying and happy.

My life has been built on a tripod:(1) I picked my parents very carefully;(2) I made a fantastic choice of a wife; and(3) I had enough sense "not to spit in my own well."

As a result, these later years are the frosting on a delicious cake that represents an amazing adventure for a young boy who started in the West End of Glens Falls as a first-generation American. In the beginning, I never dreamed that life would be so good to me. As much as the historian in me enjoys thinking and writing about the past, it is the anticipation of another day of fulfillment that makes me happy when I go to bed at night and when I arise in the morning.